Pharmacy Practice

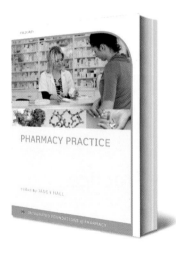

PHARMACY PRACTICE

edited by JASON HALL

INTEGRATED FOUNDATIONS of PHARMACY

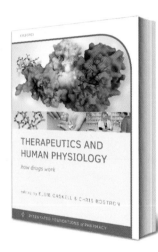

THERAPEUTICS AND
HUMAN PHYSIOLOGY

how drugs work

edited by KIRSTIE GASKELL & CHRIS ROSTRON

INTEGRATED FOUNDATIONS of PHARMACY

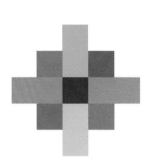

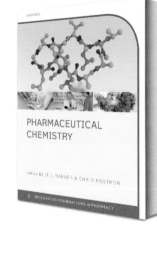

PHARMACEUTICAL
CHEMISTRY

edited by JILL BARBER & CHRIS ROSTRON

INTEGRATED FOUNDATIONS of PHARMACY

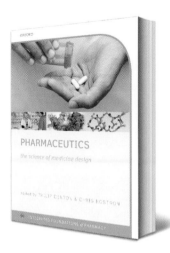

PHARMACEUTICS

the science of medicine design

edited by PHILIP DENTON & CHRIS ROSTRON

INTEGRATED FOUNDATIONS of PHARMACY

INTEGRATED FOUNDATIONS *of* PHARMACY

Pharmacy Practice

Edited by Jason Hall

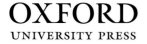

OXFORD

UNIVERSITY PRESS

INTEGRATED FOUNDATIONS *of* PHARMACY

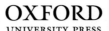

Great Clarendon Street, Oxford, OX2 6DP,
United Kingdom

Oxford University Press is a department of the University of Oxford.
It furthers the University's objective of excellence in research, scholarship,
and education by publishing worldwide. Oxford is a registered trade mark of
Oxford University Press in the UK and in certain other countries

British Library Cataloguing in Publication Data

Data available

ISBN 978–0–19–965532–8

Printed in Italy by
L.E.G.O. S.p.A.—Lavis TN

Oxford University Press makes no representation, express or implied, that the
drug dosages in this book are correct. Readers must therefore always check
the product information and clinical procedures with the most up-to-date
published product information and data sheets provided by the manufacturers
and the most recent codes of conduct and safety regulations. The authors and
the publishers do not accept responsibility or legal liability for any errors in the
text or for the misuse or misapplication of material in this work. Except where
otherwise stated, drug dosages and recommendations are for the non-pregnant
adult who is not breast-feeding

Links to third party websites are provided by Oxford in good faith and
for information only. Oxford disclaims any responsibility for the materials
contained in any third party website referenced in this work.

Preface

Integrated Foundations of Pharmacy

As a result of significant changes taking place within the profession of pharmacy there is an increasing trend for universities to adopt an integrated approach to pharmacy education. There is now an overwhelming view that pharmaceutical science must be combined with the more practice-oriented aspects of pharmacy. This assists students to see the impact of, and relationships between, those subjects which make up the essential knowledge base for a practising pharmacist.

This series supports integrated pharmacy education, so that from day one of the course students can take a professionally relevant approach to their learning. This is achieved through the organization of content and the use of key learning features. Cross references highlight related topics of importance, directing the reader to further information, and case studies explore the ways in which pharmaceutical science and practice impact upon patients' lives, allowing material to be addressed in a patient-centred context.

There are four books in the series, covering each main strand: *Pharmaceutical Chemistry*; *Pharmaceutics: The Science of Medicine Design*; *Pharmacy Practice*; and *Therapeutics and Human Physiology: How Drugs Work*. Each book is edited by a subject expert, with contributors from across pharmacy education. They have been carefully written to ensure an appropriate breadth and depth of knowledge for the first-year student.

Each book concludes with an overview of the subject and application to pharmacy, building on students' understanding of the concepts and bringing everything together. It applies the material to pharmacy practice in a variety of ways and places it in the context of all four pharmacy strands.

Pharmacy Practice

Pharmacy Practice spans a variety of areas. It introduces professionalism and looks at the origins of the profession. The roles performed by pharmacists (including prescribing, dispensing, public health, and pharmaceutical care) are covered, alongside an introduction to the structure of the health care system in the UK. Key areas such as fitness to practise; law and ethics; and how pharmacists interact with other health care professionals are explored, and we take a look at how the social and behavioural sciences play an important part in pharmacy.

Although the book is written as distinct chapters, each authored by an expert in the field, as far as possible relevant cross references have been made to related text and concepts in this book and the other books within the series. This book will provide a core understanding of the varying integrated disciplines linked to pharmacy, thus serving as a basis upon which further learning can be built.

Knowledge in the area of pharmacy practice, law, and current best practice are continuously changing. The text within this book contains drug names and relevant doses as currently prescribed, and draws on the present legislation. Readers should always consult the most up-to-date source for guidance on drug therapies and doses used, and should be constantly aware of changes to health care legislation.

Jason Hall and Chris Rostron, August 2012

Acknowledgements

The editors wish to acknowledge the support of all the contributing authors, who have spent a considerable amount of time writing and reviewing their chapters. Thanks to Sion Coulman for his support in writing Chapter 3. We would also like to extend our thanks to the staff at Oxford University Press, especially Holly Edmundson (Publishing Editor) for her continued support, encouragement, and guidance. In addition we are grateful to Jonathan Crowe, Evelyn Harvey, and Philippa Hendry for their assistance with preparing the manuscripts.

The supportive feedback from the five reviewers was greatly appreciated.

Finally, we would like to thank our past, present, and future students, who have motivated the production of this book.

Contents

8 Pharmaceutical care JASON HALL   133

An introduction to the *Integrated Foundations of Pharmacy* series

The path to becoming a qualified pharmacist is incredibly rewarding, but it requires diligence. Not only will you need to assimilate knowledge from a range of disciplines, but you must also understand—and demonstrate—how to apply this knowledge in a practical, hands-on environment. This series is written to support you as you encounter the challenges of pharmacy education today.

There are a range of features used in the series, each carefully designed to help you master the material and to encourage to you to see the connections between the different strands of the discipline.

Mastering the material

Boxes

Additional material that adds interest or depth to concepts covered in the main text is provided in the Boxes.

> **BOX 2.1**
>
> ### Bacteria versus archaea
>
> Archaea are often found living in some of the most extreme environments found on Earth, in conditions where humans would not be able to survive. These

Key points

The important 'take home messages' that you must have a good grasp of are highlighted in the Key points. You may find these form a helpful basis for your revision.

> **KEY POINT**
>
> All our cells contain identical genetic information; however the cells differentiate to make up the various types of tissues, organs, and body systems that we are made of.

Self check questions

Questions are provided throughout the chapters in order for you to test your understanding of the material. Take the time to complete these, as they will allow you to evaluate how you are getting on, and they will undoubtedly aid your learning. Answers are provided at the back of each volume.

> **SELF CHECK 1.2**
>
> Why may it be important for health care professionals to establish the family medical history?

Further reading

In this section, we direct you to additional resources that we encourage you to seek out, in your library or online. They will help you to gain a deeper understanding of the material presented in the text.

> **FURTHER READING**
>
> Boarder, M., Newby, D., and Navti, P. *Pharmacology for Pharmacy and the Health Sciences: A Patient-Centred Approach.* Oxford University Press, 2010.

Glossary

You will need to master a huge amount of new terminology as you study pharmacy. The glossaries in each volume should help you with this. Glossary terms are shown in pink.

> **ACE inhibitor**   Drug that inhibits angiotensin-converting enzyme.
>
> **Acetylcholine (Ach)**   The neurotransmitter at preganglionic autonomic neurons and postganglionic parasympathetic neurons and at the neuromuscular junction. It acts on nicotinic and muscarinic receptors. Unusually, acetylcholine is also released from sympathetic nerves that

Online resources

Visit the Online Resource Centre for related materials, including 10 multiple choice questions for each chapter, with answers and feedback.

Go to: **www.oxfordtextbooks.co.uk/orc/ifp**

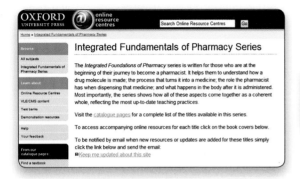

Seeing the connections

Case studies

Case studies show how the science you learn at university will impact on how you might advise a patient. Reflection questions and sample answers encourage you to think critically about the points raised in the case study.

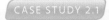

> #### CASE STUDY 2.1
>
> Angela has told Ravi she is pregnant and they are both thrilled at the prospect of being parents. However, Angela had an older brother who had cystic fibrosis (CF)

Cross-references

Linking related sections across all four volumes in the series (as well as other sections within this volume), cross-references will give you a good idea of just how integrated the subject is. Importantly, it will allow you to easily access material on the same subject, as viewed from the perspectives of the different strands of the discipline.

 The study of dosage forms is covered in the **Pharmaceutics** book within this series.

Lecturer support materials

For registered adopters of the volumes in this series, the Online Resource Centre also features figures in electronic format, available to download, for use in lecture presentations and other educational resources.

To register as an adopter, visit www.oxfordtextbooks.co.uk/orc/ifp, select the volume you are interested in, and follow the on-screen instructions.

Any comments?

We welcome comments and feedback about any aspect of the series. Just visit www.oxfordtextbooks.co.uk/orc/feedback and share your views.

About the editors

Editor Dr Jason Hall studied pharmacy at the University of Strathclyde before completing an MSc in clinical pharmacy at Liverpool John Moores University and a PhD in non-medical prescribing at the University of Manchester. He has worked in community pharmacy for 5 years, in the NHS as a pharmaceutical adviser for 2 years, and in a further education college teaching chemistry and pharmaceutical science to pharmacy technicians and science students for 5 years. Jason joined the School of Pharmacy in Manchester in 1999 and is now Director of Undergraduate Teaching and Learning. His research interests include non-medical prescribing, professional identity, and professionalism in pharmacy students.

Series Editor Dr Chris Rostron graduated in pharmacy from Manchester University and completed a PhD in medicinal chemistry at Aston University. He gained Chartered Chemist status in 1975. After a period of postdoctoral research he was appointed as a lecturer in medicinal chemistry at Liverpool Polytechnic. He is now an honorary research fellow in the School of Pharmacy and Biomolecular Sciences at Liverpool John Moores University. Prior to this he was an academic manager and then a reader in medicinal chemistry at the school. He was a member of the Academic Pharmacy Group Committee of the Royal Pharmaceutical Society of Great Britain and chairman for the past 5 years. He is currently chairman of the Academic Pharmacy Forum and deputy chair of the Education Expert Advisory Panel of the Royal Pharmaceutical Society. He is a past and present external examiner in medicinal chemistry at a number of schools of pharmacy, both in the UK and abroad. In 2008 he was awarded honorary membership of the Royal Pharmaceutical Society of Great Britain for services to pharmacy education.

Contributors

Mr Paul Duell, School of Pharmacy, University of East Anglia, UK.

Dr Dai John, Welsh School of Pharmacy, Cardiff University, UK.

Dr Joseph Bush, School of Life and Health Sciences, Aston University, UK.

Dr Sue Jones, Institute of Pharmaceutical Science, King's College London, UK.

Dr Lesley Diack, School of Pharmacy and Life Sciences, Robert Gordon University, UK.

Dr Jane Sutton, Department of Pharmacy and Pharmacology, University of Bath, UK.

Abbreviations

ACT	Accredited checking technician	IP	Independent prescriber
ADR	Adverse drug reaction	IPE	Interprofessional education
BMI	Body mass index	ISTC	Independent sector treatment centre
BNF	*British National Formulary*	MA	Marketing authorization
CD	Controlled drug	MHRA	Medicines and Healthcare products Regulatory Agency
CHRE	Council for Healthcare Regulatory Excellence	MRGCP	Membership of the Royal College of General Practitioners
CMP	Clinical management plan	MUR	Medication Use Reviews
COSHH	Control of Substances Hazardous to Health	NES	NHS Education for Scotland
CPD	Continuing professional development	NHS	National Health Service
CPPE	Centre for Pharmacy Postgraduate Education	NHSBSA	NHS Business Services Authority
CRB	Criminal Records Bureau	NI	Northern Ireland
CSM	Committee on Safety of Medicines	NICE	National Institute for Health and Clinical Excellence
DEFRA	Department for Environment, Food and Rural Affairs	NICPLD	Northern Ireland Centre for Pharmacy Learning and Development
DH	Department of Health	NMC	Nursing and Midwifery Council
DHSSPS	Department of Health, Social Services and Public Safety	*NPF*	*Nurse Prescribers' Formulary*
DPF	Dental Practitioners' Formulary	NPSA	National Patient Safety Agency
EBM	Evidence-based medicine	NRS	National Readership Survey
EEA	European Economic Area	NS-SEC	National Statistics Socioeconomic Classification
EU	European Union		
FPH	Faculty of Public Health	NVQ	National Vocational Qualification
FtP	Fitness to practise	OP	Original pack
GB	Great Britain	OTC	Over the counter
GDC	General Dental Council	P	Pharmacy medicine
GDP	Gross Domestic Product	PBL	Problem-based learning
GMC	General Medical Council	PbR	Payment by results
GNP	Gross National Product	PC	Prescriber contacted
GP	General practitioner	PCO	Primary care organization
GPhC	General Pharmaceutical Council	PCT	Primary care trust
GSL	General sale list	PIL	Patient Information Leaflet
HBM	Health belief model	PL	Product licence
HCP	Health care professional	PMH	Previous medical history
HEI	Higher education institution	PMR	Patient medication record
HLP	Healthy Living Pharmacy	PNC	Prescriber not contacted
HPC	Health Professions Council	POM	Prescription-only medicine
HRP	Household Reference Point	PSNI	Pharmaceutical Society of Northern Ireland
ICE	Ideas, concerns and expectations	QALY	Quality-adjusted life year
IFSW	International Federation of Social Workers	RCGP	Royal College of General Practitioners
ILP	Interprofessional learning provision		

RGSC	Registrar General's Social Classes	SVQ	Scottish Vocational Qualification
RPSGB	Royal Pharmaceutical Society of Great Britain	TDM	Therapeutic drug monitoring
		TPB	Theory of planned behaviour
SHO	Senior house officer	UK	United Kingdom of Great Britain and Northern Ireland
SI	Statutory instrument		
SiPPH	Specialist in pharmaceutical public health	WCPPE	Wales Centre for Pharmacy Professional Education
SOP	Standard operating procedure		
SP	Supplementary prescriber	WHO	World Health Organization
SPC	Summary of Product Characteristics		

The profession and practice of pharmacy

JASON HALL

Health care is provided by a large number of different health professionals. Patients admitted to hospital, for example, are cared for by a health care team that includes doctors, nurses, paramedics, physiotherapists, radiographers, dieticians, occupational therapists, and psychologists. Pharmacists are key members of this health care team but what is it that distinguishes pharmacists from other professions? This chapter seeks to describe what pharmacists do and considers how the pharmacy profession evolved into its current role. It will also address what being a pharmacy professional means and the social process involved in becoming a member of the pharmacy profession.

Learning objectives

Having read this chapter you are expected to be able to:

➤ Describe the roles that pharmacists perform in primary, secondary, and tertiary care.

➤ Describe the origins of the pharmacy profession.

➤ List the attributes of a profession and the benefits associated with being a professional, and discuss professional socialization.

➤ Discuss the arguments surrounding why pharmacy may or may not be considered a profession.

➤ Describe the expectations that are placed on pharmacy students and pharmacists.

➤ Describe the different professional and regulatory bodies that have an impact on the pharmacy profession.

1.1 What do pharmacists do?

The roles that pharmacists have performed have evolved over the years but the main focus of pharmacists has always been medicines. In the early days they were the experts on the preparation of medicines.

More recently pharmacists have had less need to prepare medicines as these are more often than not prepared by the pharmaceutical industry. The main aspects of the pharmacist's current role are supplying medicines and being a source of expertise on the use of medicines. Some pharmacists may be involved in both medicine supply and providing expertise on medicine use, while others may only deal with the latter.

 See 'What roles do pharmacists perform?': Primary, secondary, and tertiary care', within this section, for examples.

How do pharmacists differ from other members of the health care team?

Other professions learn about physiology, pathology, therapeutics, and medicines as well as developing their communication skills with patients, just as you will over the duration of your course, but what is it about pharmacists that makes them different? The sheer volume of training that is focused on medicines within the pharmacy undergraduate curriculum is one aspect that differentiates pharmacists from other health care professionals. No other profession devotes a comparable amount of time during the training of its practitioners to drug development and action, to medicine formulation, or to understanding a patient's behaviour towards medicines or to therapeutics.

 See Chapter 6 for more information on the skills and training that underpin the work of the other health care professionals and how their work links to the pharmacy team.

Having access to a vast knowledge base concerning medicines is important, but in today's digital world many professionals and patients are able to access the same information that pharmacists use. Therefore, what is really needed are pharmacy professionals who understand the significance of the information and who are able to apply it to the huge variety of real-life situations; this is much more challenging.

 The scientific principles you will need to progress in your course are covered in the other volumes in this series: *Therapeutics and Human Physiology*; *Pharmaceutical Chemistry*; and *Pharmaceutics*. Mastering these is fundamental to becoming a successful pharmacist.

In the past, some students have had difficulty seeing the relevance of some aspects of their scientific training to being a pharmacist practising in the community or in a hospital. The relevance was perhaps clearer for those students hoping to pursue a career in industry, but this misses the point. Understanding how a particular drug was formulated into a medicine may or may not be interesting to a pharmacy student, but the principles underpinning this knowledge are really relevant to all pharmacists. Without the science, pharmacists would not be able to explain to patients or other health care professionals why certain medicines are used in a particular way.

Understanding 'why' can aid patient education and can have a positive impact on **adherence**. For example, crystal structure and particle size may seem far removed from patient care but these have a huge impact on the rate of release of drugs from their formulation, and therefore affect timing of when the medication should be used or taken. Insulin can be formulated to be rapid acting by manipulating the crystallization of the synthetic hormone. By educating the patient as to when they should inject we can get closer to the normal physiological release of insulin in response to a meal. Other insulin formulations have been designed to release insulin more slowly over a long period of time to replicate the normal basal release of insulin.

 See Chapter 7 for more information on how the social sciences can help us to understand more about patient behaviour and see Chapter 8 for more information on adherence. More information on the structure and size of drugs, and how this affects their release rate, can be found in Chapter 2 'Solids' in *Pharmaceutics* within this series. For more information on the physiological release of insulin see Chapter 10 'This is just the beginning' in *Therapeutics and Human Physiology,* also within this series.

> **KEY POINT**
>
> A good understanding of all aspects of pharmacy—including pharmaceutical chemistry, pharmaceutics, and therapeutics—is required in order to be able to give patients the best possible advice.

In day-to-day practice, pharmacists have to evaluate scientific information. This could be when helping a patient to select a medicine to treat a minor ailment, or when determining whether a particular medicine is causing unwanted effects in a patient. Understanding definitions such as **indication, contraindication, caution, side effects** and dose can help when attempting to make sense of information in reference sources such as the *British National Formulary* (*BNF*). Frequently, however, a deeper understanding is required to put everything in context.

Problem-solving skills are often required when reviewing a patient's medical condition to determine whether the symptoms the patient is experiencing could be due to a worsening of the condition or adverse effects of the medication used to treat the condition. Once problems have been identified the pharmacist should be able to consider alternative options to overcome the problems, which could include changing the dose or formulation, switching to a different medicine, stopping the medicine, or adding another medicine to the existing medicines.

Being able to criticize, compare, and contrast evidence published in the scientific literature is an important skill that pharmacists must possess. This skill is required when attempting to determine which medicine might be the most efficacious, the safest, or easiest for the patient to take. For example, a patient or a prescriber could ask whether a recently launched medicine is safer than the medicines currently on the market. The marketing associated with the recently launched medicine may claim fewer adverse effects are associated with the new drug, but adverts can be misleading and pharmacists should be able to criticize the new evidence and produce an unbiased judgement of the evidence. Developing the skills to review and criticize evidence takes time and is a key part of the pharmacist's training.

KEY POINT

It is vital that pharmacists are able to problem solve and evaluate information so that they can feel confident that their patients are receiving the right medication based on their symptoms and the primary research available.

 See Chapter 8 for more information on developing the skills to review and critique evidence.

What specialist knowledge do pharmacists have?

- Pharmaceutical chemistry
- Biological sciences (physiology, pharmacology)
- Physical sciences (dissolution)
- Pharmaceutical sciences (medicine formulation, stability, and testing)
- Therapeutics (medicine selection, monitoring therapy)
- Behavioural sciences (medicine-taking behaviour)

What specialist skills do pharmacists have?

- Interpretation and application in practice
- Clinical skills
- Pharmaceutical problem-solving skills

SELF CHECK 1.1

What skills, other than those already listed, do you think pharmacists should have?

What roles do pharmacists perform?

There are nearly 40 000 pharmacists in Great Britain and around 2000 in Northern Ireland. The majority (around 70%) work in community pharmacy. Hospital pharmacy accounts for the second highest proportion with around 20% of pharmacists being employed in that sector. Much smaller numbers of pharmacists are employed in industry, academia, and primary care.

Primary, secondary, and tertiary care

Primary care is usually the first point of contact a patient has with the health services although there are exceptions, such as visiting the accident and emergency department of a hospital. Primary care includes general practices, dentists, optometrists, and community pharmacists. General practices contain physicians known as general practitioners (GPs) and frequently employ practice nurses; they may occasionally also employ a pharmacist. Patients requiring further care, such as invasive examinations or surgical operations, may be referred by their GP to a hospital (secondary care). A relatively small proportion of patients may have to be referred to a specialist centre for further treatment, such as a cancer hospital (tertiary care).

 See Chapter 2 for more information on the organization of health care in the UK.

Community pharmacies, also known as chemist shops, have both a supply and a medicines information role. They provide pharmaceutical services to the general public without an appointment or the need for the patient to register with the pharmacy. The supply role includes dispensing prescriptions and selling over-the-counter (OTC) medicines (see Figure 1.1). The role of the pharmacist as medicines expert includes advising patients on medicines use, reviewing a patient's medicines, treating minor ailments, and screening for poor health.

The community pharmacy team consists of pharmacists, pharmacy technicians, and pharmacy assistants. In Great Britain the term pharmacy technician is a protected title and all those who wish to use this title must have a competency-based qualification (National Vocational Qualification [NVQ] Level 3 or Scottish Vocational Qualification [SVQ] Level 3) and a knowledge-based qualification, and must also have completed the appropriate period of work experience prior to registration with the General Pharmaceutical Council (GPhC). Pharmacy assistants who work on

FIGURE 1.1 A community pharmacist preparing a patient's prescription.
Source: © Lloyds Pharmacy, 2012. Reproduced with permission

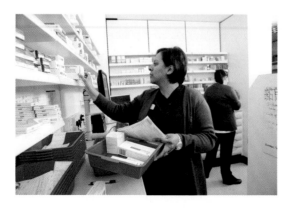

the medicines counter must have, or be working towards completing, an accredited medicine counter assistant's course. Pharmacists must be registered with the GPhC.

Pharmacists have also been employed by general practices and in National Health Service (NHS) primary care organizations (PCOs) since the early 1990s to support the work of the general practice in providing expertise on medicine use without supplying medicines. In this role they may review the medicines that have been prescribed for individual patients to ensure that their conditions are effectively treated and that they are not experiencing any adverse effects. Some pharmacists have been trained to prescribe and may prescribe medicines for patients they see in the clinic. They can also provide advice to GPs on appropriate prescribing. Pharmacist in PCOs may also perform a public health role, advising on the pharmaceutical health needs of the population.

 See Chapter 4 for more information on public health.

The pharmacy team in secondary and tertiary care is composed of pharmacists, pharmacy technicians, pharmacy assistants, and clerical staff (Figure 1.2). As within primary care, pharmacists and pharmacy technicians in Great Britain must be registered with the GPhC. Pharmacists perform a wide variety of roles in secondary and tertiary care in the NHS and private hospitals; these include supply, clinical services, and provision of information. Some pharmacists are generalists and cover all the common medical treatments, while others, especially those in tertiary care, may specialize and focus on a narrow range of medicines. There are also different grades of pharmacist working in secondary care in the NHS, starting with junior pharmacists (Band 6), and moving up to clinical pharmacists (Band 7), and then chief pharmacists and consultant pharmacists (Band 8).

The hospital pharmacy service provides a supply role, dispensing medicines to patients who are staying in the hospital (inpatients) and also to patients who may just be attending a clinic in the hospital (outpatients). This supply role may be performed by pharmacists and/or pharmacy technicians. Pharmacists in some hospitals

FIGURE 1.2 The hospital pharmacy team.
Source: © South Tees Hospitals NHS Foundation Trust, 2012. Reproduced with permission

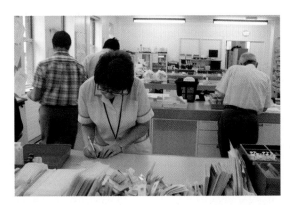
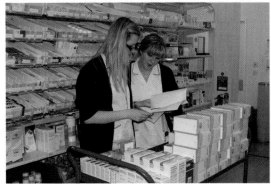

5

may specialize in the manufacture of pharmaceuticals. Examples of pharmaceuticals prepared in hospital include sterile medicines such as injections, intravenous nutrition for patients unable to take food through the gastrointestinal system, and radiopharmaceuticals used in imaging or cancer therapy.

Many hospital pharmacists will perform a clinical role and will visit patients on the wards to discuss the selection and monitoring of medicines. As experts on medicine use they will advise other health care professionals on the use of medicines in the hospital. Some hospital pharmacists may be able to prescribe medicines for patients. Some pharmacists may specialize in an area of therapeutics such as haematology, cardiology, or diabetes or may specialize in the care of the very young (paediatrics) or the very old (geriatrics). Medicine (or drug) information is a pharmacy specialization in which pharmacists with access to an extensive range of information on drugs and medicines are available to advise hospital staff and health care workers outside the hospital.

Academia

Pharmacists are also employed in academia in a teaching and research capacity. All schools of pharmacy in the UK are required by the GPhC to employ an appropriate number of pharmacists to contribute to the teaching of pharmacy undergraduates. This is to ensure that a student's education and training are relevant and that they prepare the student to join the profession. Significant numbers of the pharmacists who teach in schools of pharmacy split their time between

academia and practice, such that they may spend 2 or 3 days per week teaching in the university and the rest of the week working in a community or a hospital pharmacy (teacher practitioners).

Pharmacists are also engaged in all aspects of pharmaceutical research, but not all who conduct such research are pharmacists. Many staff engaged in pharmaceutical research within a school of pharmacy are not pharmacists. Such staff bring expertise from a variety of fields, which helps to strengthen the research and teaching profile within the school. Pharmaceutical research includes research in the physical, chemical, and biological sciences as well as the social and behavioural sciences. The traditional sciences cover drug molecule development, dosage forms, drug action (how the drug works on animals or humans), and drug handling (how the body deals with the drug). The social and behavioural sciences deal with how professionals and patients act and the organization of health care services. Many of the pharmacists involved in research will have studied for a higher degree such as a PhD.

 See Chapter 7 for more information on the involvement of the social and behavioural sciences in pharmacy.

Pharmaceutical industry

Pharmacists are employed alongside other scientists in many different sectors of the pharmaceutical industry. A pharmacy degree is likely to provide students with an awareness of each of these sectors and the breadth of pharmaceutical training that a pharmacist receives can be an advantage. However, pharmacists will be competing for jobs in industry with those who may have more specialist knowledge and skills because they have focused on a narrower range of scientific disciplines.

The companies which comprise the pharmaceutical industry range from the very small, employing perhaps up to 50 people, right up to multinational companies employing several thousand people. The nature of the work they perform also varies a great deal. Some companies are at the cutting edge and invest heavily in developing new medicines in addition to developing and marketing their existing portfolio of branded medicines. Other companies may limit their production to generic medicines, which are medicines that are no longer covered by a **patent** and can be made and sold more cheaply by other companies (see Box 1.1).

 See Chapter 5 for more information on prescribing.

The development of new medicines includes the development of new drug molecules; this traditionally has involved scientists with expertise in pharmaceutical chemistry. Investigating how and where drugs act in the body involves knowledge of pharmacology. An important area for the development of new medicines is the identification of new targets within the body for drugs to act on. Once suitable drug molecules have been identified they must be formulated into a medicine; formulation scientists with expertise in the science of pharmaceutics will develop the new medicinal formulation and test its stability.

New medicines must undergo rigorous testing to ensure they are safe and effective. Pharmacists can work alongside physicians and nurses during the clinical trial stage of developing a new medicine. There are different types of clinical trials:

- Phase 1 clinical trials involve testing the drug in a small number (20–100) of healthy volunteers to determine the drug's safety and what the body does to the drug (**pharmacokinetics**), and to describe what the drug does to the body (**pharmacodynamics**).

- Phase II clinical trials involve a larger number of patients (several hundred) and explore how effective and safe the drug is.

- Phase III clinical trials are larger still and may contain thousands of patients. The purpose of this phase is to further establish how effective the drug is compared with other therapies.

Even when a product is launched onto the market, companies will continue to invest in clinical trials to collect further evidence regarding the safety and efficacy of their medicine. The ongoing safety of medicines is also monitored via the yellow card system (Figure 1.3), whereby health professionals and patients report suspected adverse drug reactions to the Medicines and Healthcare products Regulatory Agency (MHRA).

 See Chapter 8 for further information on the MHRA.

BOX 1.1

Generic and brand names

Losec® is the brand or trade name given to the medicine containing the drug omeprazole. Losec® is manufactured and marketed by AstraZeneca. As the patent covering omeprazole has expired it can now be manufactured and sold by other companies. For example, Bristol Laboratories manufactures 'generic' omeprazole.

A branded medicine has two names: the brand name and the generic name. The brand name starts with a capital letter whereas the generic starts in lower case. Thus Losec® is the brand name and omeprazole is the generic name.

A generic medicine usually has only one name. However, confusingly, some manufacturers of generic medicines create a new brand name for their generic medicine. The new brand name must be different from the original.

When prescribing and dispensing, the name written on the prescription form is important:

- If the brand name is written on the prescription then that branded medicine must be dispensed.

- If the generic name is written on the prescription then the branded medicine or the generic medicine can be supplied.

FIGURE 1.3 A poster from the Medicines and Healthcare products Regulatory Agency to raise patients' awareness of the yellow card system. *Source:* © Crown Copyright 2009

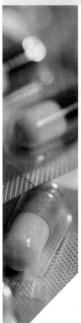

YellowCard *

Helping to make medicines safer

A side effect to a medicine?

You can report it using
YellowCard *

Visit **www.mhra.gov.uk/yellowcard** to report suspected side effects

You can get Yellow Card forms:
● from pharmacies or GP surgeries
● by calling 020 3080 6764

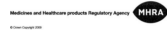

Medicines and Healthcare products Regulatory Agency **MHRA**

© Crown Copyright 2009

Before a medicine can be marketed to prescribers (or patients if it is an OTC medicine) it must have been issued with a marketing authorization (previously a product licence) from the MHRA. The authorization indicates that the medicine has met the appropriate standards of safety, quality, and efficacy. Pharmacists can work in licensing alongside the company's legal team to compile the evidence required to obtain the marketing authorization.

Medicines in the UK are generally allocated to one of three major legal classifications depending upon the restrictions placed on their sale or supply:

- *POM*: Medicines which require a prescription are termed prescription-only medicines.

- *P*: Medicines which can be sold in a pharmacy under the supervision of a pharmacist are termed pharmacy-only medicines.

- *GSL*: Medicines which can go general sale in a retail outlet without a pharmacist's supervision are termed general sale list.

 Details of medicine types are elaborated in Chapter 5.

The quantities of medicine required for the clinical trial stage are relatively small and companies must scale up to produce sufficient quantities for commercial manufacturing. The quality control procedures in place during manufacturing and storage of the medicines must ensure that the medicine complies with the appropriate quality standards and is safe. The quality control laboratory will test samples from each batch to ensure that the medicine is of the appropriate quality. Failure of samples to meet the appropriate standard could pose a risk to patient safety and would result in recall of the batch. It would also have major cost implications for the company and could possibly harm its reputation.

Pharmaceutical companies invest heavily in marketing so that prescribers and patients are aware of the benefits of their medicines. Marketing includes activities such as advertising and visiting prescribers. Representatives from the pharmaceutical company (drug reps) visit prescribers and provide them with information on their company's medicine. They will usually try to show that their medicine is either more effective, easier to take, safer, or cheaper than alternative medicines on the market. Pharmacists can be involved in either the training of the company representatives or could be one of the representatives.

KEY POINT

Pharmacists working in primary, secondary, or tertiary care are responsible for, among other things, dispensing medicines, monitoring therapy, and advising patients and health care professionals on all matters pertaining to medicines. Within academia, pharmacists are responsible for teaching and research. Those pharmacists working in the pharmaceutical industry will be involved in developing new medicines, testing them in clinical trials, and marketing them once they are approved.

1.2 **Historical development of the health professions**

Being a member of a profession brings a range of benefits, which include status and standing within the community, job security, and salary. If we were to ask members of the public why they think health professionals occupy an elevated position in society they may well say it is because they help save lives or that people rely on them when they are in need. Modern medical interventions can certainly help to save lives but there was a time when medical interventions such as blood-letting were more likely to do harm than good. However, even when medical interventions were of doubtful benefit at best, the health professionals still had a high social standing. To understand why this is we must take a look back at how the professions have developed. Many of these developments have been political rather than being based on scientific advances in health care.

Origins of pharmacy

Some of the earliest traders to sell medicines and other items such as herbs and spices to the public were apothecaries. The word apothecary is derived from *apotheca,* which means the place where wines, herbs, and spices are sold. In general the wealthy would have consulted physicians regarding their health and the apothecaries would have dispensed the medication prescribed by the physician. The less well off would have consulted apothecaries then purchased the medications they recommended. Unlike the physicians, apothecaries derived their income from the sale of the medicines rather than charging a fee for a consultation.

In the early part of the second millennium, craftsmen and traders around towns formed livery companies or guilds, which attempted to form monopolies so that only their members could sell their products to people in the town. At this time there were few towns such as would be recognizable today, and much of the early development happened in London, with developments spreading out to other areas much later. Pharmacy followed a slightly different evolutionary path in Scotland and Ireland. In London, the earliest sellers of products for medicinal uses belonged to guilds such as the Guild of Pepperers, the Guild of Spicers, and later on the Worshipful Company of Grocers. Many merchants selling drugs and spices sold their products by wholesale or *en gros,* which is probably where the name grocer originates.

In 1617 James I of England (James VI of Scotland) signed a charter that established the Worshipful Society of the Art and Mystery of the Apothecaries in London. This allowed the apothecaries to split from the grocers and created a monopoly for apothecaries in London as it restricted the keeping of an apothecary shop to members of the society. It also gave the society the right to inspect and examine those who had completed an apprenticeship, which lasted a minimum of 7 years. It did not prevent other retailers, such as the chemists and druggists (who did not have to complete any training at this point in time), from selling drugs, medicines, or poisons. In many ways the seventeenth-century apothecary may appear similar to the modern-day community pharmacist in that they dispensed prescriptions issued by physicians and sold medicines from shops. In many countries in Europe apothecaries evolved into pharmacists. The word for pharmacy in German is *apotheke* and in Danish it is *apotek.* However, in the UK apothecaries evolved along different lines.

Eighteenth and nineteenth centuries

In the eighteenth and nineteenth centuries there were many battles between the physicians and the apothecaries regarding who was encroaching on whose area of practice. In 1704 the apothecaries won a legal battle with the physicians in the House of Lords regarding the right to prescribe and dispense medicines, which was an important step in the evolution of apothecaries as they moved closer towards the practice of medicine. Apothecaries performed a slightly different role in Scotland. Selling medicines formed a large part of the role of most Scottish apothecaries but some also performed minor operations. Practising surgeon–apothecaries were incorporated into the Royal College of Surgeons of Edinburgh in 1778.

There was a massive increase in the wealth of the population during the eighteenth century, which led to a retail revolution as a greater proportion of the population were able to purchase items that previously could only have been purchased by the very wealthy. This increase in commercial activity coincided with a demise in the guild system of restricting who could practise and a huge growth in retail businesses, including the chemists and druggists. The chemists and druggists were not part of the guild and they took advantage of the favourable commercial environment.

It was not always easy to distinguish between an apothecary and a chemist and druggist. A defining characteristic of the chemists and druggists was the shop; many of them invested in the retail side of their business, creating attractive eye-catching window displays with giant jars (carboys) of brightly coloured water. Apothecaries generally had a shop attached to their laboratory and consultation room. Apothecaries also visited patients in their homes on occasion, while chemists and druggists did not leave their shops.

The unregulated nature of chemists and druggists caused concern regarding the quality of dispensing, products sold over the counter, and the sale of poisons (Figure 1.4). Several bills were proposed to parliament that would have brought the chemists and druggists under the control of physicians and apothecaries. Under such bills the physicians and apothecaries would have been responsible for examining chemists and druggists at the end of their apprenticeship and would also have had the power to inspect their premises.

In 1841 a bill was published that sought to reform the practice of medicine. This bill would have prevented chemists and druggists from being able to advise patients or recommend products for purchase. A group of leading chemists met to raise objections to the bill, which failed to progress through lack of support in the House of Commons. The chemists and druggists nonetheless realized that the lack of control regarding who could operate as a chemist and druggist was a threat to all their futures. These leading chemists formed the Pharmaceutical Society to raise

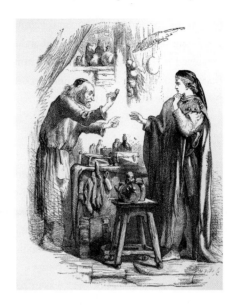

FIGURE 1.4 In Shakespeare's *Romeo and Juliet*, Romeo buys poison from the apothecary. Illustration from *The Illustrated Library Shakespeare*, published London 1890. *Source:* ©Ken Welsh / The Bridgeman Art Library

the standing of the profession and to protect the interests of its members. The society was granted a charter from Queen Victoria in 1843.

In 1858 there was a public outcry following the accidental poisoning of 200 people in Bradford, which resulted in 20 deaths. The poisoning was caused by a chemist and druggist incorrectly supplying arsenic for use in peppermint lozenges. The government sought to impose controls over the sales of poisons to prevent such accidents from happening in the future. The Pharmaceutical Society was criticized for opposing these controls, which would have improved safety. The society opposed the bill because it focused only on poisons and the society wished to have control over a wider range of chemists' and druggists' activities, including dispensing. Legislation in 1858 led to apothecaries in England joining physicians in being governed by the General Medical Council. English apothecaries therefore evolved into GPs. Apothecaries in Ireland also occasionally performed surgery and they joined surgeons to become Registered Medical Practitioners.

Almost 20 years after the Bradford poisonings the Pharmaceutical Society won the right in 1868 to register chemists and druggists. In addition, those wishing to join the register in the future would have to pass the society's exam (see Figure 1.5 for a summary of changes to pharmacy education over the years). In the early days, membership of the Pharmaceutical Society was restricted to men. Women were allowed to sit the exams but were not allowed to become members of the society. The situation regarding membership was finally resolved in 1879 following the admittance of two women to the register, but it was another 40 years before women were elected to the council.

Twentieth century

At the end of the nineteenth century in England and Wales the majority of dispensing was carried out by the prescribing physicians themselves. In Scotland and in much of the rest of Europe at this time chemists and druggists carried out a much greater proportion of the dispensing of physicians' prescriptions.

The National Insurance Act of 1911 was introduced by David Lloyd George when he was Chancellor of the Exchequer. This was a compulsory insurance scheme for those earning below a certain limit and was funded by contributions from the employee, the employer, and the government. It allowed employees who contributed to the scheme to receive free medical treatment. This Act separated the roles of prescribing and dispensing, which set the scene for the rest of the twentieth century.

The government believed there was a conflict of interests in physicians writing prescriptions and making a profit by dispensing their own prescriptions. The physicians were originally opposed to losing the ability to dispense their own prescriptions but their opposition faded when they realized they could maintain or increase their income from the consultation payments. The Pharmaceutical Society also negotiated with the government to ensure that dispensing was carried out by those who were qualified. Following implementation of the 1911 Act it became illegal for someone other than a chemist or druggist to dispense prescriptions issued by a physician. Physicians could dispense their own prescriptions in rural locations if there was no chemist and druggist available, and this practice exists to the present day. However, it was not illegal for an unqualified person to sell any medicine at this time.

During the First World War, concern over the abuse of cocaine by soldiers led to the first drug restriction, such that this and a small number of other drugs could only be supplied in response to a prescription issued by a physician. This restriction expired at the end of the war but, shortly after, the Dangerous Drugs Act of 1920 was passed, which brought similar restrictions.

The partitioning of Ireland in the 1920s into Northern Ireland and Southern Ireland (later the Republic of Ireland) also divided the pharmacy profession. In 1925 the Pharmaceutical Society of Northern Ireland (PSNI) was formed and took over responsibility for regulating the pharmacy profession in the province.

In 1948 the NHS was formed, having been devised by Aneurin Bevan. This had a major impact on the provision of medical and pharmaceutical services in the UK. For the first time the entire population were

FIGURE 1.5 Timeline of pharmacy education

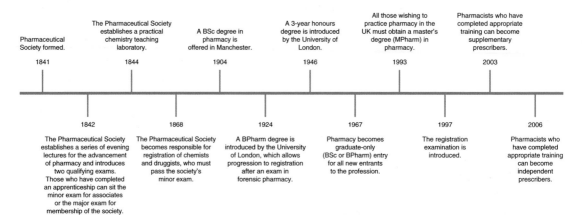

able to receive free medical treatment and free medicines, although prescription charges were introduced for some patients in 1952. There was a tremendous demand for these free medical services. Previously, pharmacists had spent a great deal of their time advising patients on medical matters and selling products over the counter. The introduction of free medical advice from physicians and free medicines (at least in the early days of the NHS) meant that pharmacists spent less time advising patients and more time dispensing NHS prescriptions. Pharmacists were paid a fee to dispense each item on a prescription. As all their NHS income was derived from dispensing there was little incentive to develop other clinical services from the community pharmacy.

 See Chapter 2 for more information on the development and structure of the NHS.

Towards the end of the twentieth century the role of the pharmacist evolved further. The hospital pharmacist's role extended with the development of specialist clinical services, with pharmacists visiting patients on the wards and becoming closely involved in treatment decisions. In the mid-1980s services developed in community pharmacy included giving advice to care homes and promoting better health. These extended roles have continued, with the addition of medication reviews and supervised administration of medicines for drug misusers. More recently, the development of 'pharmaceutical care' has led to a shift towards the patient being the focus of the pharmacist's attention. This is a radical change in role as pharmacists take responsibility for achieving outcomes that will improve patients' quality of life, rather than just supplying medicines.

 See Chapter 8 for more information on pharmaceutical care.

Twenty-first century

In 2003 legislation was passed that allowed a pharmacist with sufficient experience, and who had successfully completed the appropriate training programme, to become a **supplementary prescriber**. Supplementary prescribers can prescribe any

Independent prescriber requirements

There are two requirements that registered pharmacists must meet to become independent prescribers:

1. *Training*: The programme comprises a minimum of 26 days at a higher education institution, although some of this could involve distance learning, plus 12 days 'learning in practice' supervised by a designated medical practitioner.

2. *Experience*: Pharmacists are required to have a minimum of 2 years' post-registration experience.

medicine, provided it has been agreed with a medical prescriber and specified in a **clinical management plan (CMP)** prepared for the patient. In 2006, further legislation was passed that allowed a pharmacist who had successfully completed the appropriate training (see Box 1.2) to become an **independent prescriber**, who can prescribe most drugs without needing a CMP. Most training programmes for pharmacists wishing to prescribe cover both supplementary and independent prescribing. The learning outcomes and indicative content for both are very similar, but there are additional requirements covering diagnostic and clinical assessment associated with independent prescribing.

The Pharmaceutical Society has undergone name changes and role changes in the last 30 years. In 1988 the Queen granted the title of Royal Pharmaceutical Society of Great Britain (RPSGB). In 2010 the society was effectively split into two organizations. The regulatory role became the responsibility of the GPhC. The GPhC provides a similar role for pharmacists to the General Medical Council (GMC) for medical practitioners and the General Dental Council (GDC) for dentists. The renamed Royal Pharmaceutical Society became the professional leadership body for the pharmacy profession in Great Britain.

KEY POINT

The role of pharmacists has developed over hundreds of years. Throughout history a key theme has been their focus on medicines.

1.3 **Attributes of the professions and benefits of being a professional**

The term 'professional' is commonly used in different ways. It can be used to describe someone who receives payment for an activity, such as a professional footballer. It is also used to describe a member of a profession (for example, medicine, dentistry, law, and of course, pharmacy), which is how it will be used in this book. This section will explore why people want to join a profession, and also what sets professions apart from other occupations.

Entry to the professions is via successful completion of a period of education, usually in a higher education institute. Some professions require an additional period of training. In general, there is greater competition for entry to university degree programmes that are required for entry to a profession than for those that are not. To understand why there is greater competition we must consider what differentiates the professions from other occupations. Members of the professions have a status in society that is reflected in the social class they are allocated to in the UK national census (they were previously assigned to social class I and are now assigned to subgroup 22 in skill level 4).

 See Chapter 4 for more information on social classification systems.

Professionals generally occupy managerial positions in the organizations in which they work. The work that professionals undertake could be considered to be more rewarding, challenging, and interesting, which could be because such people are in control of their own workload to a greater extent (see 'Autonomy' in this section). In general, unemployment rates in the professions are lower than among other occupations, which is partly due to the monopolies that exist. The lower rates of unemployment and shortages of professionals have generally resulted in higher salaries for those registered with a professional regulator.

Attributes of a profession

There are many occupations that are associated with higher levels of remuneration, and some may also have a certain status in society, but they are not necessarily all classed as professions. What is it that makes a profession different from other occupations?

Knowledge

Professionals have access to specialized information that is often not available or understandable to those outside the profession. Obviously, there are many occupations that require the possession of specialized knowledge; what distinguishes that used by a member of a profession is the balance between technical knowledge (which is available in textbooks, manuals, or online) and indeterminate knowledge (all the other knowledge required to process the technical knowledge). For example, a textbook on neurosurgery may provide details on the technical procedure involved in brain surgery but it is highly unlikely that any lay person would have sufficient indeterminate knowledge to perform the procedure.

Monopoly

The professions generally have a monopoly over who can perform their professional role. There are restrictions regarding the use of professional titles. It would be an offence to mislead people by claiming to be a medical doctor or a dentist if you were not registered with the appropriate regulator (the GMC or the GDC). In the UK, only those who are registered with the GPhC or the PSNI are entitled to call themselves a pharmacist. It would be an offence for anyone else to call themselves a pharmacist.

Many roles can only be performed by those registered with the appropriate regulator. Until relatively recently the only professions able to prescribe medicines for human use were doctors and dentists. The sale or supply of medicines other than those on the general sale list can only be carried out from registered pharmacy premises; other retail outlets cannot compete with community pharmacies regarding the sale of pharmacy-only or prescription-only medicines. Therefore pharmacists operate a monopoly with regards to the selling of medicines in the UK. It is important to realize that there are some countries where this monopoly does not exist and anyone can open a pharmacy and sell medicines.

 See Chapter 3 for more information on the General Sale List.

Autonomy

Members of professions operate with autonomy, which means they are in control of the work that they do—they do not require their work to be checked or authorized by someone else. Professions also regulate themselves. Originally the councils that regulated each profession were composed entirely of members of that profession. Now, the regulators all have lay members as part of their governing council. Pharmacists are regulated by the GPhC, which is composed of pharmacists and lay people.

Service orientation

Professionals must put the interests of their clients or patients before their own. All members of a profession are bound by a code of ethics. The code should guide the professional in their work.

SELF CHECK 1.2

How does a community pharmacist differ from other high-street retailers in terms of professionalism?

KEY POINT

Professionals can be defined as those with access to specialized information and a monopoly over who can perform their role. They operate with autonomy and are bound by a code of ethics.

Is pharmacy a profession?

We shall consider the arguments for and against pharmacy being considered a profession under each of the four attributes of a profession (see Table 1.1).

TABLE 1.1 Arguments about pharmacy as a profession

Attribute	For	Against
Knowledge	• Although some products can be purchased for minor ailments without any professional input there can be problems for patients with other conditions who are taking other medications. • It is often difficult to differentiate between a minor ailment and something more serious without objective professional advice. • The assessment of comorbidities and potential drug interactions, and ascertaining the severity of a condition, all require indeterminate knowledge.	• The knowledge required to select and dispense medicines is largely technical and is readily available to the lay public. • Many medicines are now available to purchase from supermarkets and other retail outlets so it is not necessary visit a pharmacy.
Monopoly	• Many medicines are still only available from a pharmacy. • Prescriptions can only be dispensed by a pharmacy or a dispensing doctor (if in a rural location). • 'Pharmacist' is a restricted title.	• The availability of some medicines from other retail outlets and the availability of information online to patients have reduced the monopoly of pharmacists.
Autonomy	• Pharmacists do not require their work to be checked by any other professional. • Pharmacists are regulated by the General Pharmaceutical Council, which is governed by pharmacists and lay people in a similar arrangement to the other health professions.	• The major part of a pharmacist's work involves dispensing prescriptions. In this role they are working under the direction of the prescriber, who is most likely to be a doctor.
Service orientation	• Pharmacists are bound by a code of ethics that makes the care of patients their first concern. • A proportion of a community pharmacy's income is derived from the provision of additional services, which are paid for at a flat rate in a similar manner to other professions.	• The majority of pharmacists are employed in community pharmacies where they sell their products. It is in their interests to sell more medicines and thereby increase their profits.

SELF CHECK 1.3

What do you think about the arguments in Table 1.1? Discuss these arguments with your friends or tutors. You may find other criteria or have your own ideas with which to justify pharmacy being considered a profession. What do you think are the threats to the future status of pharmacy?

 See Chapter 8 for a discussion of the future professional status of pharmacy.

1.4 Becoming a health professional

Before you started on a pharmacy programme you would have been considered a lay person. After successfully completing the MPharm degree and the pre-registration period you will be eligible to register with the regulator (GPhC or PSNI) and be entitled to call yourself a pharmacist. Moving from being a lay person to a qualified professional is a big change. Not only will you have gathered a considerable amount of knowledge and developed a wide range of skills, but your attitudes and values may well also undergo a major change. This change is called professional socialization and it describes how a lay person evolves into a member of a profession.

The first stage of professionalization happens during selection. The selection will involve submitting an application form, attending an interview and possibly completing additional tests. Applicants have to indicate why they wish to study to become a member of that profession. If the reasons given during the application procedure do not adhere to the values and norms of that profession then the application could be rejected.

Entry to most professions follows after successful completion of a programme at a higher education institute and, in some cases, a period of supervised practice. In most cases the programme of study at the higher education institute takes place in a specialized school such as a school of medicine, school of nursing, school of dentistry, or school of pharmacy. The school structure can have a major impact on professional socialization. Traditionally in most schools the students study their chosen profession in isolation from other students, especially in the later years of the programme. There have been attempts in recent years to promote interprofessional learning by encouraging students from different disciplines to work and learn together about each other's roles in addition to learning about patient care. Such initiatives are to be applauded but nevertheless a major part of the undergraduate education is delivered in isolation from students on other programmes.

Professionalism is covered in the formal curriculum and is also addressed informally during interactions between students and staff. The knowledge and skills that are required by the profession are described in the formal curriculum and will be covered in lectures, tutorials, practical classes, and work placements. The knowledge and skills may be formally assessed. The values, attitudes, and behaviours that the profession expects will become apparent to students when those staff who are also members of the profession discuss the practice of pharmacy. These aspects may not be formally assessed but students may be more likely to reflect these values, attitudes, and behaviours because they assume they are required or believe they will enhance their prospects.

Professional socialization does not necessarily end with graduation. Employers will select graduates who can demonstrate the appropriate professional attributes for pre-registration training. Similar selection will occur when seeking employment as a pharmacist and when being considered for promotion within an organization.

What is expected of professionals?

In return for the benefits associated with being a member of a profession, which have been described above, there are a number of expectations that society places on health professionals. The public expect health professionals to:

- apply a high degree of skill and knowledge to their work;
- act in the best interests of patients and the public and not be influenced by self-interest;
- be objective and non-judgemental;
- be guided by the standards of their profession.

In pharmacy the standards that must be adhered to are produced by the GPhC. The GPhC is the independent regulator for pharmacists and pharmacy technicians in Great Britain. In Northern Ireland the PSNI fulfils this role for pharmacists. The GPhC have produced standards (Box 1.3) which pharmacists must follow in their practice. These standards cover a number of areas of practice.

 See Section 1.5 for more on regulation.

See Section 1.5 for more on regulation.

BOX 1.3

GPhC *Standards for Conduct, Ethics, and Performance*

The standards that pharmacy professionals must follow consist of seven principles:

1. Make the care of patients your first concern
2. Exercise your professional judgement in the interest of patients and the public
3. Show respect for others
4. Encourage patients to participate in decisions about their care
5. Develop your professional knowledge and competence
6. Be honest and trustworthy
7. Take responsibility for your working practices.

Fitness to practise

Pharmacists must act professionally at all times. It is important to realize that the responsibility to act professionally extends beyond the pharmacy workplace into all areas of life. Anything that could have a negative impact on an individual's ability to be an effective and safe practitioner or on the confidence the public have in the profession could impair fitness to practise.

A lack of adherence to the standards published by the GPhC is one area that could raise fitness to practise concerns. Engagement in unlawful behaviour could compromise public confidence in the profession and could therefore impact upon an individual's fitness to practise. This means they could face a fitness to practise hearing in addition to any penalty that the courts may impose. For example, if a pharmacist were found guilty of possessing illegal drugs while out socializing they could receive a fine from the courts and also be struck from the register of pharmaceutical chemists for bringing the profession into disrepute.

A pharmacist's poor health can also affect their fitness to practise. Contagious diseases could put patients and colleagues at risk. Poor mental health could impact on a pharmacist's judgement, compromising their ability to work effectively and safely. Pharmacists have a duty to seek and follow advice from a suitably qualified professional about their health.

KEY POINT

Pharmacists must act professionally at all times, in both their personal and professional lives.

What is expected of pharmacy students?

In 2010 the *Code of Conduct for Pharmacy Students* was published by the GPhC and adopted by the PSNI. It applies to all students studying pharmacy in Great Britain and Northern Ireland. It is based upon the same seven principles in the GPhC *Standards of Conduct, Ethics, and Performance*. This code applies to pharmacy students from the first day of their course and covers all that they do even while they are away from their school of pharmacy. Students' behaviour on and off the programme can have a major impact on their ability to progress through the MPharm programme and ultimately register as a pharmacist.

Schools of pharmacy in the UK are required to have fitness to practise procedures in place to consider students when their fitness to practise is in doubt. The primary aim of these procedures is to protect the public and maintain public confidence in the profession. The GPhC has published *Guidance on Student Fitness to Practise Procedures in Schools of Pharmacy*, which covers the scope of fitness to practise, the threshold of fitness to practise, the range of outcomes, and the key elements in fitness to practise proceedings.

In addition, schools of pharmacy must consider the fitness to practise of applicants to the MPharm programme. Attracting applications from across all sectors of the community is important if the composition of the pharmacy workforce is to reflect the population it serves. Students with a wide range of backgrounds, health conditions, and disabilities can be accommodated on the MPharm programme, but students must be able to achieve the learning outcomes. The learning outcomes cannot be altered, but reasonable adjustments could be made to the method of assessing the learning outcomes for a student with health problems or disabilities. However, the safety of patients must be the priority and MPharm students must be fit to practise pharmacy.

SELF CHECK 1.4

Why do you think pharmacy students must be fit to practise?

1.5 How is pharmacy regulated and supported?

The Pharmaceutical Society's role in regulating and supporting the advancement of pharmaceutical knowledge has been described in the historical development section.

In 2010 the regulatory function was separated from the professional support function in Great Britain. The GPhC was created to fulfil the regulatory function, while the Royal Pharmaceutical Society of Great Britain began to focus purely on professional development and changed its name by dropping the reference to Great Britain. The splitting of the regulatory and professional roles did not occur in Northern Ireland, where the PSNI retains both roles.

The regulator's role is 'to protect, promote and maintain the health, safety and well-being of members of the public by upholding standards and public trust in pharmacy'. It performs this role by setting standards for conduct, ethics, proficiency, education and training, and continuing professional development (CPD), and taking action where standards are not being met (see Section 1.4 for a discussion of the standards or see the GPhC website for the full list of standards). The regulator is responsible for maintaining the register of pharmacists. Only those who are on the register are eligible to call themselves pharmacists. There is only one register of pharmacists in Great Britain and one in Northern Ireland although entries in the register can be annotated to show additional qualifications, such as being an independent or supplementary prescriber. The regulator also maintains a register of all retail pharmacy premises. The regulators have inspectorates, who visit registered premises to ensure that they are complying with relevant legislation and professional standards.

The regulator has established fitness to practise requirements for pharmacists. It has a duty to deal fairly and proportionately with complaints and concerns about a pharmacist's fitness to practise (see Section 1.4). If a complaint is received from a patient, a member of the public, or another health care professional then the regulator's inspectors may investigate the complaint. If the investigation finds that there is evidence of impaired fitness to practise then the matter will be heard by the GPhC Investigating Committee. This meets in private to consider all the evidence presented to it and can decide to refer the matter on to the Fitness to Practise Committee. The Fitness to Practise Committee holds its meetings in public unless the hearing concerns the health of the registrant. The committee can call witnesses. If it is found that a registrant's fitness to practise is impaired then it may: issue a warning, issue a direction to remove a registrant's name from the register, issue a direction to suspend a registrant from the register, or issue a direction that states the conditions which the registrant must comply with to remain on the register.

The regulator must approve qualifications for pharmacists and accredit education and training providers. Pharmacy degree programmes in the UK must be accredited by the regulator every 6 years. In Great Britain the GPhC is the sole regulator and in Northern Ireland programmes are jointly accredited by the PSNI and the GPhC. The standards by which the programmes are accredited can be found on the GPhC's website.

> **KEY POINT**
>
> Regulators uphold standards and public trust by ensuring that all those working within the profession are adhering to the appropriate professional standards. They also handle complaints and concerns about a pharmacist's fitness to practise.

Professional bodies

The Royal Pharmaceutical Society is the professional body for pharmacists in Great Britain. The PSNI is the professional body and the regulator for pharmacists in Northern Ireland. The aim of the professional body is to promote pharmacy and to advance science, practice, and education in pharmacy. Membership of the professional body is not a requirement to practise in Great Britain but is needed in Northern Ireland as the regulator and professional body are joined. Membership of the Royal Pharmaceutical Society is open to pharmacists and retired pharmacists. Those working in an area related to drug or medicine development, use, or education are eligible to become pharmaceutical scientist members. Pharmacy students are eligible to become student members. Student members will also receive joint membership of the British Pharmaceutical Students Association. Membership of the PSNI is restricted to pharmacists.

Pharmacists can also become members of additional bodies, which represent different branches of the profession. These bodies exist to promote the interests of the branch they represent and also provide additional support such as continuing education and professional indemnity insurance. Membership of these bodies is not a requirement to practise in an area. The National Pharmacy Association is the community pharmacy trade body representing the interests of its members. The Guild of Healthcare Pharmacists (previously the Guild of Hospital Pharmacists) represents the interests of individual employed pharmacists working in hospitals, primary care, and other health care institutions within both the NHS and commercial health care providers throughout the UK.

Each of the home nations of the UK has an organization providing support for CPD for pharmacists working in the NHS, which includes community pharmacists. In England this is provided by the Centre for Pharmacy Postgraduate Education, and in the other parts of the UK it is provided by NHS Education for Scotland, Wales Centre for Pharmacy Professional Education, and Northern Ireland Centre for Pharmacy Learning and Development.

> **CHAPTER SUMMARY**

➤ Pharmacy students spend a greater proportion of their time focusing on the science and practice of medicine preparation and use compared with other health care professionals.

➤ The majority of pharmacists work in primary and secondary care as members of the pharmacy team providing both a medicine supply role and expertise on medicines use.

➤ The origins of pharmacy can be traced back to the medieval times with the foundation of town guilds.

➤ The pharmacist's right to dispense medicines was firmly established with the passing of the National Insurance Act in 1911. The dispensing role became an even greater part of the pharmacist's role with the introduction of the NHS in 1948.

➤ The four attributes associated with the professions are knowledge, monopoly, service orientation, and autonomy.

➤ Being a member of a profession brings several benefits but there are also obligations associated with membership. Members of professions are expected to apply a high degree of skill and knowledge to their work, act in the best interests of patients and the public, be objective, and be guided by the standards of their profession.

➤ Pharmacy students must abide by the *Code of Conduct for Pharmacy Students*. Failure to comply with this code could result in a student's fitness to practise being called into question.

➤ In Great Britain the regulator for pharmacy is GPhC and in Northern Ireland it is the PSNI.

FURTHER READING

Anderson S. *Making Medicines: A Brief History of Pharmacy and Pharmaceuticals*. Pharmaceutical Press, 2005.

This book provides a history of pharmacy from the ancient world through medieval times up to the end of the twentieth century. There are chapters focusing on the development of community pharmacy, hospital pharmacy, pharmacy education, and the pharmaceutical industry.

General Pharmaceutical Council. *Code of Conduct for Pharmacy Students*. GPhC, 2011.

All pharmacy students in the UK should receive a copy of the code. It contains the seven principles that apply to pharmacy students and provides guidance as to how the principles apply to students.

Royal Pharmaceutical Society. *Medicines Ethics and Practice: The Professional Guide for Pharmacists*. RPS, 2011.

This guide aims to support pharmacists in their day-to-day practice when they are faced with decisions to make.

Medicines and Healthcare products Regulatory Agency. *Pharmacovigilance: How we Monitor the Safety of Medicines*. MHRA, 2012. <http://www.mhra.gov.uk/Safetyinformation/Howwemonitorthesafetyofproducts/Medicines/Pharmacovigilance/index.htm>.

This brief guide explains the role of the MHRA in monitoring the safety of medicines. Elsewhere, the website provides an overview of the MHRA's licensing and authorization functions.

Organization of health care in the UK

PAUL DUELL

The process of providing health care for the whole population is complex and requires significant financial investment. This chapter will give an overview of how the current system was developed and will start to explain how it is financed and managed at national, regional, and local levels. The importance of the quality of care provided by professionals is a major factor in how organizations are created and maintained. The impact of this within pharmacy is considered using the concept of clinical governance to demonstrate what this means for practising pharmacists.

Learning objectives

Having read this chapter you are expected to be able to:

➤ Describe how health care is funded in the UK.

➤ Recognize the roles of independent contractors within health care provision.

➤ Define the inter-relationships between primary, secondary, and tertiary care.

➤ Describe the function of National Health Service (NHS) organizations and bodies.

➤ Identify the importance of local health care professionals' involvement with commissioning for the local population.

➤ Recognize the reasons why the structure of the NHS changes frequently.

➤ Define the key principles of clinical governance.

➤ Identify how quality is monitored throughout the NHS.

➤ Recognize the importance of quality within pharmacy services.

2.1 The creation of the NHS and its impact on service provision

Prior to the creation of the NHS in 1948, access to health services was limited and was dependent upon individuals being able to pay, being covered by National Insurance (see Chapter 1), or having access to charity. Consequently, those who were not working, many elderly people, and the families of workers were denied treatment or relied on home remedies. Those who could afford to pay for their medicines could get the local pharmacist to dispense their prescription or could purchase a proprietary product or a chemist's nostrum (a product made by the pharmacy). The full cost of the prescribed medication was paid for by the patient. Pharmacists were often the only health care professionals accessed by patients, which gave them an important role within primary care provision.

The birth of the NHS on 5 July 1948 suddenly granted free access to health care to the whole population. Family practitioner services were created. Doctors, dentists, opticians, and pharmacists entered into a contractual relationship with the government to provide specific services for which the government paid the costs instead of the patients. The contractual arrangements allowed the health care professionals to remain as independent contractors and to continue to provide additional services to patients outside the NHS framework. The NHS, at this time, also started to pay for hospital services.

The first NHS prescriptions were free to all, and as a consequence the number of prescriptions quickly grew, from 70 million per year pre-NHS to over 240 million per year by 1950. There was also a steep drop in the number of proprietary medicines and chemists' nostrums sold. Demand for all health services rapidly increased, far in excess of what the government of the day had anticipated, as patients used the new opportunities to address long-standing health problems. The medicine cost alone in 1948 was £18 million.

The government's role in NHS funding and health care monitoring

The post-war labour government anticipated that the creation of the NHS would put additional pressure on the tax system but believed that the concept of free health care at the point of need to all, regardless of wealth, was vital. Two other major determinants of health—housing and a balanced diet—were also affected by the war. There was food rationing and a major shortage of housing while rebuilding took place in bomb-damaged cities.

It very quickly became clear to the government that the NHS was consuming more financial resources than had been anticipated and that services were not being targeted based on need. The monitoring of health care outcomes against spend was from the outset an important government function, and plans were devised to try and control more effectively how and where the funds were spent. As early as 1952 the government introduced prescription charges of one shilling (5p) and a flat rate of £1 for dental charges in order to reduce demand and curtail rising costs.

Aneurin Bevan, the first health secretary, anticipated that 'we shall never have all we need' and that expectations would always exceed capacity. He also believed that the service must always be changing, growing, and improving, and that it would always appear inadequate. The task in hand would be about balancing resources and demands to get the best possible outcomes. This is as true today as it was in the early days of the NHS, and all the governments in between have modified the systems and processes in order to try to maintain this balance.

There are a number of factors that continue to put pressure on the NHS budget. These include technological advances that create better or new forms of treatment; new drug treatments for previously unmanaged or poorly controlled conditions; increased life expectancy; greater patient expectation; increase in the population owing to the birth rate exceeding the death rate and because of immigration; and more professionals with new or expanded roles.

Comparison of spending on the NHS is often conducted in economic terms by considering the cost as a percentage of the country's gross domestic product (GDP). GDP is a measure of the total economic activity occurring in the UK. Since the early 1960s NHS spending as a proportion of GDP has increased from 3.5% to 8.0% (in 2009). It must be borne in mind that GDP is not a fixed figure, it constantly changes, so this is not an absolute growth in spending—it is just a comparator of how the government's resources are allocated on a year-on-year basis.

Providing free health care requires carefully balancing resources and demands to get the best possible outcomes. Advances in medical science mean that we are now living longer and have higher expectations of what medicine can do. Managing these increasing demands is a constant challenge for the NHS.

Why is the number of prescriptions issued each year in England still rising?

Major differences between England and the rest of the UK

In each of the constituent parts of the UK the terminology describing different parts of the health care structure may differ, and there may also appear to be differences regarding the management of services. However, the overall structure is similar, with the state funding the vast majority of care via NHS-managed services in primary, secondary, or tertiary locations. Primary care consists of GP practices, district nursing, pharmacies, dental surgeries, and optometry practices. Secondary care comprises hospitals; tertiary care is very specialized care within hospital settings and could be, for example, specialized cancer treatment centres.

 See Chapter 1 for more information on the role of pharmacists in primary, secondary, and tertiary care.

In England and Wales the strategy and legal framework for health care is set by the Department of Health. There are some differences between England and Wales due to the Welsh Assembly setting their own modifications. An example of this would be the provision of free NHS prescriptions for patients in Wales whereas charges still exist in England. In Scotland, the Scottish Government Health and Social Care Directorate and the regional NHS boards implement the priorities set by ministers. In Northern Ireland, the Department of Health, Social Services and Public Safety (DHSSPS) was created in 1999 to improve the health and social well-being of the people of Northern Ireland. The DHSSPS is responsible for health and social care policy and legislation, public health, and public safety, which includes fire and rescue services.

How funding is distributed

Each of the constituent parts of the UK has its own mechanism for allocating NHS funding to different services and localities. These mechanisms take into account the priorities of the governing administration and involve an allocation formula to distribute the budget. These formulae are based on historical funding and take into consideration the population size and demography, with greater weightings applied to elderly or disadvantaged people. Further information on how the devolved administrations in Northern Ireland and Scotland allocate their budgets can be found on the administrations' websites.

 See the 'Further reading' section for links to the health department sections of the websites of the Northern Irish and Scottish administrations.

Nearly 80% of the NHS budget in England is managed within primary care, with the remaining 20% spent in secondary or tertiary care. Although 80% is managed within primary care, a large percentage of this money is spent on purchasing care from secondary and tertiary care providers. The Department of Health uses an allocation formula to distribute the budget across the country via regional and local NHS commissioning organizations. GP practices or GP lead groups are becoming more influential in how the funding is managed locally. Until April 2013, strategic health authorities act as the regional bodies that, on behalf of the Department of Health, ensure that the budgets allocated to local areas via primary care trusts (PCTs) or hospital trusts are properly managed and monitor expenditure so that budgets are not exceeded.

 For a description of PCTs see Section 2.3 'Local NHS organizations'.

The government has worked out set prices for many hospital services and procedures, which are known as the tariff price. This is sometimes referred to as the payment by results (PbR) tariff. This allows hospitals to work out their potential income by predicting the amount of activity they can provide. It also allows the body that commissions services to understand the cost of providing those services to its patients.

Over the last few years the government has put processes in place to ensure that the people involved with spending NHS resources and commissioning NHS services to meet service demands (the commissioners), are not also directly responsible for providing those services. This has meant that PCTs, who employed all the health visitors and school nurses and managed district hospitals, have had to stop doing so. New organizations have taken over all these services and managed them independently of the PCTs.

The government over the last decade has allowed more private health companies to tender for NHS work or has bought capacity from private companies to improve waiting times for busy services. So although these services are accessed from private providers they are still funded as part of the NHS system.

So far, we have only discussed health care that is provided by the state. There have always been private companies or organizations that have provided health care to those who are willing to pay for the service or those who have an insurance scheme that covers the cost of their treatment. Nowadays, many employers offer free private health cover or free health insurance to their employees as a company perk. This health care cover may not cover every condition or treatment and the patients may still find themselves accessing some services via the NHS or having to pay additional amounts to cover the gaps in costs.

KEY POINT

Health care can be provided by the NHS or private companies. In some cases the NHS uses private companies to deliver NHS services.

Prescription charges

Patients who are receiving private treatment will receive a private prescription for any medication they require. They have to pay for these medicines and the cost may well be a lot higher than that of an NHS prescription. NHS prescriptions are free to:

- children aged under 16 years;
- young people aged between 16 and 18 years in qualifying full-time education;
- people aged over 60 years;
- those with a valid exemption certificate (see Box 2.1);
- those receiving income support, income-based jobseeker's allowance, or income-related employment and support allowance;
- war pensioners holding a valid war pension exemption certificate for prescriptions;
- those who have purchased a prescription prepayment certificate.

BOX 2.1

The criteria for an NHS prescription exemption certificate

There are several valid criteria for an NHS prescription exemption certificate. These include women who have borne a child or women who have given birth to a child in the last 12 months and patients with:

- a permanent fistula (colostomy, laryngostomy, ileostomy, caecostomy) requiring continuous surgical dressing;
- a form of hypoadrenalism for which specific substitution therapy is essential;
- diabetes insipidus and other forms of hypopituitarism;
- diabetes mellitus, except where treatment is by diet alone;
- hypoparathyroidism;
- myasthenia gravis;
- myxoedema (hypothyroidism requiring thyroid hormone replacement);
- epilepsy requiring continuous anticonvulsive therapy;
- a continuing physical disability which means they cannot go out without the help of another person;
- cancer.

Patients must complete the back of the prescription, as shown in Figure 2.1, indicating the reason why they are exempt from the charge and must sign to confirm that the information is correct. Many types of prescription have been used so far (see Chapter 5), but the declaration form printed overleaf is still the same. The pharmacy that dispenses the prescribed medicine is responsible for collecting any prescription charges that are due from patients who are not exempt.

Patients in England who are not exempt from NHS charges and receive two or more prescription items each month are better off having a prepayment certificate.

A prescription prepayment certificate can be purchased by anyone who does not meet any of the other exemption criteria or if the prescription is not for a

FIGURE 2.1   The prescription form. This must be completed by all patients collecting their prescription.

NOTE Patients who don't have to pay must fill in parts 1 and 3 (unless they are exempt on age grounds, and their age is printed on the front of this prescription). Those who pay must fill in parts 2 and 3. Penalty charges may be applied if you make a wrongful claim for free prescriptions. If you're unsure about whether you are entitled to free prescriptions, pay and ask for an FP57 form. You cannot get one later. The FP57 tells you about getting a refund.

Part 1   The patient doesn't have to pay because he/she:

Collectors of Schedule 2 & 3 CDs should sign their name:

A   ☐ is under 16 years of age
B   ☐ is 16, 17 or 18 **and** in full-time education
C   ☐ is 60 years of age or over
D   ☐ has a valid maternity exemption certificate
E   ☐ has a valid medical exemption certificate
F   ☐ has a valid prescription pre-payment certificate
G   ☐ has a valid War Pension exemption certificate
L   ☐ is named on a current HC2 charges certificate
X   ☐ was prescribed free-of-charge contraceptives
H   ☐ *gets Income Support or **income-related** Employment and Support Allowance
K   ☐ *gets **income-based** Jobseeker's Allowance
M   ☐ *is entitled to, or named on, a valid NHS Tax Credit Exemption Certificate
S   ☐ *has a partner who gets Pension Credit **guarantee** credit (PCGC)

pharmacy use only
Evidence not seen

*Name: | Date of Birth: | NI no:

* I am included in an award of **income-based** Jobseeker's Allowance, **income-related** Employment and Support Allowance, Income Support, Pension Credit Guarantee Credit or Tax Credit. **Print** the name of the person who gets the benefit.

Declaration *For patients who do not have to pay*
I declare that the information I have given on this form is correct and complete. I understand that if it is not, appropriate action may be taken. I confirm proper entitlement to exemption. To enable the NHS to check I have a valid exemption and to prevent and detect fraud and incorrectness, I consent to the disclosure of relevant information from this form to and by the NHS Business Services Authority, the Department for Work and Pensions and Local Authorities.

Now sign and fill in Part 3

Part 2   I have paid | £ | Now sign and fill in Part 3

Part 3   *Cross ONE box* I am the patient ☐   patient's representative ☐

Sign here ✍ | Date   /   /

Print name and address* |
   | Postcode

*If different from overleaf   © Crown Copyright

James Vickers receives free private health care from his employer. His wife, Rachel, works as a teacher in Manchester. They have three children: Miriam (aged 5), Maya (aged 3), and Joseph (aged 6). Rachel's mother Naina is staying with the Vickers family during the school holidays. She has diabetes mellitus.

The whole family get an infection and go to see their doctor. Mr Vickers goes to see the doctor employed by his company and the rest of his family go to see their local NHS GP. All are issued with a prescription for antibiotics and Mrs Vickers takes them all to her local pharmacy.

The cost of Mr Vickers' prescription, which will be covered by his private health care, is £19.69.

REFLECTION QUESTIONS

1. Which members of the family will have to pay for their prescriptions?

2. Why does Mr Vickers' prescription cost more than Mrs Vickers'?

Answers

1 Mrs Vickers will have to pay the charge of £7.65 for her prescription. The three children are all under 16 and therefore exempt from payment. Mrs Vickers' mother is also exempt from paying as she has a valid exemption certificate owing to her diabetes. Mr Vickers has been supplied with a private prescription and his employer will have to pay the full cost.

2 Mrs Vickers has to pay the standard prescription fee irrespective of the cost of the item. This cost will not vary between pharmacies. The cost of Mr Vickers' prescription is dependent on the cost of the medicine prescribed and also where it is dispensed. Each pharmacy sets its own private prescription fee. Some may add a percentage to the cost of the item whereas others may add a set fee. Theoretically, a private prescription could cost less than an NHS prescription if the drug cost is very low but some pharmacies set a minimum fee, which could be equal to the NHS fee.

contraceptive drug. The certificate can be bought to cover a period of 3 months or 1 year. The price of these certificates usually increases each year, as does the prescription charge.

The prescription charge has increased significantly since its introduction in 1952. In April 2012 the prescription charge was £7.65. The extensive number of exemptions, along with the prepayment process, means that today the prescription charge is no longer used to try and reduce prescription numbers and is seen purely as a tax to offset the NHS's expenditure on drugs. Case Study 2.1 reviews private and NHS prescriptions and who pays for their NHS prescriptions.

2.2 Health care provision

Primary care

General practitioners

When anyone is asked to define primary care the likelihood is that the definition will predominately focus on general practitioners and GP practices. There are many reasons for this close association, which include the social status associated with local doctors and their role as gatekeepers to accessing more specialized health care. For many patients their local doctor is still their first port of call for any health-related matter or concern. Most GP practices have significantly expanded from the days when they consisted of a lone GP with perhaps some administrative assistance.

The skill of GPs involves diagnosing medical conditions, assessing the most relevant treatment required, and identifying where that can be best obtained. The development of a practice team around the GP has created an environment in which many diagnostic tests and treatments can now be provided within the practice by practice staff. This has given the practice a more patient-focused approach and helped to reduce more expensive secondary care referrals. Over the last decade, governments have strongly supported having larger practices, with more GPs working together, as this provides economies of scale, the sharing of best practice, and peer support for doctors. The latter point is thought to be particularly beneficial for patient safety following high-profile cases where lone practitioners such as Harold Shipman (who was found guilty of murdering 15 patients) were allowed to work in isolation from colleagues.

When the NHS was created, GPs were allowed to become independent contractors. This meant that although the vast majority of their work comes from the NHS they are not prevented from providing additional non-NHS medical services. Although they are bound to comply with the terms of their NHS contract they are not directly employed by the government and hence they are free to manage their business in the way they see fit. This means that if the government wants to significantly change the way primary care is provided they have to get the buy-in of GPs. This independent contractor status helps to give GPs their current level of influence on the management of primary care because it is recognized that they are the main change catalysts.

The second most widely recognized health care professionals in primary care (and secondary care) are nurses. The expansion of GP practices has created more opportunities for nursing staff to take on different roles, with some **practice nurses** being supplementary or independent prescribers. Supplementary prescribers can prescribe medicines or appliances, provided they have been specified on a clinical management plan, whereas independent prescribers can prescribe almost all medicines. However, both supplementary and independent prescribers should restrict prescribing to medicines within the area of their own competency.

 See Chapter 1 for more information on supplementary and independent prescribers.

Practice nurses can have a particular area of specialization and run clinics in the practice, for example as an asthma nurse. Other practice nurses include nurse practitioners, who have the ability to manage patients and make their own decisions. Practices also often employ health care assistants, who do not have a nursing qualification but act as assistant nurses, helping to care for patients.

GP practices can employ a range of other professionals, such as speech and language therapists, **phlebotomists**, dieticians, mental health workers, social workers, and physiotherapists. Increasingly, pharmacists work in the practice, either when a pharmacy is located within the practice or as a practice pharmacist.

Some GP practices may directly employ health visitors or district nurses, but these professionals are more likely to be employed by a community trust or social enterprise. These are not-for-profit health organizations. Health visitors are registered nurses or midwives who have undergone additional training. They work in a variety of settings, including GP practices and patients' homes, and usually cover a geographical area. District nurses also cover a geographical area and work in different locations, including GP practices. District nurses are also qualified nurses, who have at least 1 year's additional training that gives them specialist practitioner training. School nurses provide health and sex education and health screening, and administer immunizations.

 See Chapter 6 for more information on the range of health care professionals a pharmacist will work with.

GP practices are allocated a prescribing budget. This is worked out based on historical spending and, like the allocation of the rest of the NHS expenditure, is adjusted to match the practice population characteristics. In general, elderly patients take three times as many medicines as younger patients, and patients living in areas of high socioeconomic deprivation receive a greater number of prescribed medicines. That means that if two practices were to have the same number of patients, the practice with a higher proportion of elderly patients or a higher proportion of patients living in deprived areas would be allocated a larger drugs budget. Each month, information on medicines and appliances prescribed by the practice is collected via community pharmacies reporting to the appropriate pricing organization. The cost of the items on the prescriptions is calculated and reported back to the GP practice so they can see how they are performing against their budget.

See Chapter 5 for more information on prescribing.

See Chapter 5 for more information on prescribing.

> **KEY POINT**
>
> The budget available to GP practices to spend on pre-scribing depends on the age and socioeconomic back-ground of their patients.

In rural areas, where it is not viable to run a community pharmacy, some GPs are allowed to dispense as well as prescribe medication—known as dispensing doctors. There are different regulations and there is a different contract for dispensing doctors from those for community pharmacies.

Pharmacists

Community pharmacists are also independent contractors. There are over 12 000 community pharmacies in the UK (approximately 10 000 in England, 1200 in Scotland, 700 in Wales, and 500 in Northern Ireland). The owner of the contract can be a small, medium, or large company or an individual or partnership. The core contract for a community pharmacy requires the pharmacy to open for a minimum of 40 hours per week. The number of pharmacies in the country is controlled. Complex regulations set the criteria for applying to open a new pharmacy, and these have to be met along with demonstrating why a new pharmacy is needed. Special panels are set up to review each application and decisions can be legally challenged.

Approximately 90% of a community pharmacy's income comes from the NHS, which is in contrast to the general perception that community pharmacies are predominantly retail businesses. In 2005 the community pharmacy contract in England was changed. Services were classified as being essential, advanced, or enhanced. All pharmacies have to provide essential services, but advanced and enhanced services are optional. Essential services include dispensing medicines, repeat dispensing, signposting, public health, waste management, supporting self-care, and clinical governance. Advanced services are those that have been designed at national level and have set criteria and payment mechanisms. An example of an advanced

service is a medicines use review, where pharmacists carry out structured adherence-centred reviews with patients on multiple medications. Enhanced services are commissioned locally and can vary from area to area. They can include needle exchange services, supervised administration of prescribed medication, and care-home support.

Dentists

Dentists can work privately, work fully for the NHS, or in a combination of the two. If they carry out any work on behalf of the NHS they work as an independent contractor. Just over half the English population receives NHS dental treatment. This is a big decrease from the early days of the formation of the NHS. This has been predominantly due to dentists preferring private work to the NHS contract, as the NHS contract has fewer funding incentives. A new NHS dental contract was created in 2006 that changed the basis on which payments were made. The contract now measures units of dental activity. There are different bands of activity depending on the type of work carried out.

Optometrists

Optometrists can have a general ophthalmic service contract to provide NHS services and can be independent NHS contractors. This contract covers preventative and corrective eye care for children, people aged over 60, people on low incomes, and those that have a predisposition to or are suffering from eye disease. In 2010 in England and Wales 12.5 million eye tests were provided on the NHS and £204 million was spent on optical vouchers to provide glasses.

> **SELF CHECK 2.2**
>
> Who are independent contractors?

Secondary care

Foundation trusts

In England only, the government has created foundation trusts. In the rest of the UK NHS trusts exist. This change in England was made to give the public a much greater say in how the trusts operate. Members of the public who live in the area covered by a trust, and its staff, can become members of the organization. Members over the age of 16 can stand to be elected onto the board of governors. They receive regular information on the trust and have an opportunity to respond to plans for future developments and services.

Foundation trusts differ from other trusts in that they have greater operational and financial freedom. NHS organizations differ from the private sector in that any savings made against the budget cannot be carried over into the next financial year and have to be returned to the government. Foundation trusts are treated more like private companies and are allowed to spend any savings.

An organization called Monitor has been set up to oversee the effective financial management of foundation trusts. The role of Monitor will change over the coming years, with further expansion planned to ensure providers of health care comply with quality standards.

The government has indicated that all hospital trusts in England should aspire to become foundation trusts as soon as it is clinically feasible, so that the public can have a greater influence on the running of health care. Some hospital trusts are teaching trusts. There is no single definition of a teaching trust but many are linked to schools of medicine and provide practical training for medical students and newly qualified doctors. There are still a number of small district general hospitals in towns around the country, which provide a range of services close to where patients live. In some cases they are managed by larger hospital trusts or foundation trusts. Some are run by community health trusts or social enterprises. The range of services available is limited and more complex cases are usually referred to larger hospitals.

Independent sector treatment centres (ISTCs) are another way in which additional capacity and choice is added to the NHS. They specialize in treating specific conditions rather than providing the full range of services that are found in most hospitals. The companies that run these centres are privately owned and financed and they enter into a contract to provide NHS services. A criticism of this system is that the ISTC business model is based on providing only services that are seen to be profitable whereas a traditional hospital will provide a wide range of services that may be expensive to provide. It is suggested that ISTCs can threaten the viability of existing hospitals.

Tertiary care

Tertiary care is provided in specialized NHS-owned centres. It is particularly useful for very rare conditions and diseases for which treatment cannot be provided in local hospitals owing to either a lack of expertise or the very high costs associated with providing the treatment. Tertiary centres can provide high-quality care because of the centralization of the service and they often lead the research in treating and managing rare conditions.

2.3 **The structure of the NHS**

The structure of the NHS is extremely complex, as could be expected of a system that employs 1.4 million people and has a budget of £90 billion. The simplest way to start to get an understanding of how all the organizations, bodies, and groups fit together is to consider them separately at three levels, from national, regional, and local perspectives. A grasp of the horizontal and vertical integration of these bodies will begin to map out the inter-relationships.

National NHS organizations

The complexity of the NHS has grown owing to the need to manage, monitor, and provide more services to more patients. A general increase in life expectancy has meant that there is a greater need for continued care over a longer time period; some patients, for example, may be living with an illness for over 80 years. In addition, as patients live for longer the likelihood of having **comorbidities** increases. Added to this is the greater expectation that the NHS will keep us healthier for longer and has the ability to significantly reduce the complications and symptoms of numerous conditions.

Why do we have national health-related organizations and bodies?

Central coordination is essential if there is to be any consistency in how health services are provided. Patients expect that they should all get consistently high-quality services at a time and a place that is convenient to them. Standardization of treatment processes, outcomes, and waiting times reduces significant local variation but leads to a perennial NHS dilemma: if all monitoring and all decisions are made nationally then it is easier to get a unified consistent service but what might suit the needs of a population in a rural location might be completely different to what is needed by people living in a deprived inner city.

If there were to be only local management systems then these would be able to alter priorities to address local issues and needs. This is more patient-focused and responsive. However, this creates increased costs and can lead to huge variation in access and quality. So what should the government do? In reality most governments tend to have a favourite position and prefer either a central or local approach. However, they tend to create a mixture of the two, with a greater emphasis on their preferred style. Governments that prefer a centralist approach tend to have more national organizations overseeing service delivery whereas governments that prefer greater local accountability have more local systems to support health care.

Who are they and what patient benefit do they provide?

In England, the Department of Health is the government body that has the responsibility for delivering the NHS and implementing the current government's health plans and reforms. The chief executive of the Department of Health is directly accountable to the Secretary of State for Health. In Scotland, the Scottish Government Health and Social Care Directorate and the regional NHS boards implement the priorities set by

ministers. In Northern Ireland, the DHSSPS is responsible for implementing health and social care policy. New government policies often require a fundamental change in the structure of NHS organizations in order to deliver the new agenda, improve efficiencies and outcomes, or reduce costs. The bodies within the respective administrations oversee these changes and review their effectiveness in meeting their new roles.

Monitoring NHS expenditure and assessing service outcomes is conducted by the respective body for each part of the UK, which also prioritizes future spending. In England, the monitoring role follows a traditional line-management process, with regional NHS organizations being directly accountable to the Department of Health and local organizations being accountable to the regional bodies.

Other national organizations have more specialized roles that encompass a particular sphere of importance to the NHS. Among these are bodies called special health authorities. These are independent organizations that can still be subject to ministerial direction. The name comes from an older NHS structure where regional and local health organizations were referred to as health authorities. Special health authorities cover the whole of England; the National Blood Service is an example of this. It provides a unified approach to a service that can be managed centrally. The requirements of the service are consistent across geographical areas so it is consequently more efficient to have one joined-up system rather many local organizations providing exactly the same function.

There are a large number of national organizations whose functions are specifically related to collating evidence and sharing best practice, areas of focus include clinical treatments and management. Such organizations include the **National Institute for Health and Excellence (NICE)** and **Scottish Intercollegiate Guidelines Network (SIGN)**. Other organizations have the function of monitoring the quality of health care provision and regulating the providers of health care. Monitor is the largest of these organizations and has the responsibility for regulating NHS secondary care providers and other NHS trusts. The **National Patient Safety Agency (NPSA)** is responsible for ensuring that there is a coordinated approach to protecting patient safety, that lessons are learnt from previous incidents, and that this information is shared to minimize the risk of the same mistake happening again in another area.

The national organizations that have been considered so far are related to general health care provision. One of the reasons for the complexity of the NHS structure is the number of organizations that exist at each level. Each organization has different functions and relates to either different population groups or covers a specific area of health care. There are consequently a large number of national organizations that specifically deal with matters relating to pharmacy. Some are from a whole-profession perspective whereas others focus only on community or hospital or primary care.

 See Chapter 1 for details of some of the national organizations relating to pharmacy.

Regional NHS organizations

As the population of England is very much greater than in the other parts of the UK there is a need to group localities together into regions. The regional NHS organizations in England are currently known as strategic health authorities; there are 4 of these, a decrease from a high of 28 regions.

Regional health bodies can be seen as a true compromise between a centralist approach and a locality-based one. There is still a sharing of functions between a number of organizations, and consistency can be provided over a bigger geographical area. However, the region can also accommodate local variation. At this level the management is not seen as too distant by patients and clinicians because it is more accommodating of local needs. There may also be a common bond between local organizations that are used to dealing with similar issues in their localities and often work together on cross-boundary services.

Local NHS organizations

The geographical size of the local NHS organizations has changed frequently. Currently, the local NHS organizations in England are the PCTs. These are accountable to the strategic health authority for the commissioning of services. Health care managers work with local health care professionals to decide on commissioning priorities and to consider how services could be provided more effectively and efficiently. GPs have a central role within this process and it is intended that this will become more formalized with local clinical commissioning groups taking over the role of PCTs by 2014.

Public involvement

Public and voluntary groups can work at any of the three levels. Voluntary groups tend to be more localized and represent the needs of patients and their carers in the vicinity of service provision. Having an effective patient voice in the commissioning of services is important, so local groups play a vital role. The government supports the creation of local, regional, and national groups to provide a public perspective to health care, and mandates local health organizations to actively engage with these patient groups. The naming of the groups and their method of operation changes very frequently, but the concept remains that patients need to be part of the design and modification of health care services.

Another key way that the public is involved in health care is the appointment of lay members to the boards of health organizations. The board normally consists of more non-executive directors (who are not clinicians) than executive directors (NHS employees or clinicians) and the board chair is a lay member. The appointment of non-executive directors is carried out by another national NHS organization.

Why does the structure of the NHS change so frequently?

Throughout the history of the NHS there has been constant change in the structure of how its services are delivered and managed. This goes beyond changes caused by new treatments and organic development. In part this comes from Aneurin Bevan's philosophy that the NHS should always be adapting, changing, and improving. It is also due to the fact that the NHS remains a national institution and reflects the public perception of the quality of the government that is in power at that time.

Consequently, the impact of UK politics has significantly shaped the development of the NHS. Every opposition party believes they can manage the NHS better and improve outcomes for patients while improving value for money. Thinking has to be innovative as new policies cannot be a copy of existing or old polices. Changing organizational structures and procedures clearly demonstrates a different way of working and produces change management processes. Major change is not restricted to changes in government. Governments that are in power are constantly monitoring the success of their new structures and are mindful of the need to prove to the electorate the improvements they have made. Change has to be visible within the life of a parliament so it has been a common occurrence for structures to change midway through a government's period of office. The extent of the change is driven by the government's perception of how slowly change is occurring. Another reason for midterm change is unforeseen changes in health care or economic decline.

We have already discussed the perpetual need to improve efficiency and quality and to control costs. There is also a constant drive to evaluate organizational structures, which is also found in all businesses outside the NHS. This type of developmental change is always occurring, only occasionally involves wholesale change, and occurs at different speeds in different organizations.

The process of change management within a system as big as the NHS is very difficult. The analogy is often made of the NHS being a supertanker. Getting it to change direction does not happen immediately; it requires time. An issue for any change management programme is how do the decision makers persuade the workers to change their practice and adopt the new ways of working? An added complication within the NHS is that the front-line workers are clinical professionals who have their own professional autonomy when treating patients. The need for clinical engagement is therefore something that all governments have tried to address. Failure to get the clinicians on

board will prevent even the best of plans from coming to fruition.

The election of the coalition government in May 2010 brought about another period of massive NHS reorganization. The extent of the change is so large that it will probably not be until 2014 that the bulk of the changes have taken effect. Many of the structures will change but the core principles behind the changes have already been discussed. The NHS will continue to have the three tiers previously described—at national, regional, and local levels—with a greater focus this time on localities driving clinical change. In particular, GPs are expected to be the prominent leaders. In keeping with the model of local and regional decision-making, the number of national organizations is set to decrease.

The key strategic change that differs from anything that has gone before is the move to delegate to the independent NHS Commissioning Board many of the functions that were previously carried out by the Department of Health. It will be responsible for ensuring that all local decision-making groups are performing their roles effectively and maintaining standards. It will use regional groups to help monitor performance and delivery in a similar way to existing structures. Making the NHS Commissioning Board independent is meant to reduce the amount of political control of the NHS. However, the Secretary of State for health continues to be ultimately responsible for the NHS.

The public health functions carried out by the Department of Health will be taken over by a new body called Public Health England. This is in recognition of the growing importance of preventing ill-health rather than just focusing on treatment. Public Health England will work closely with local and regional groups to target public health advice to the needs of the local populations.

The second fundamental change is the desire for greater integration between the NHS and social care. Many determinants of poor health are social factors such as poor education and housing and unemployment. Bringing the two sectors closer together should have economic as well as health benefits. Consequently, local authorities will have a much greater role in the decision-making regarding the local provision of health care, with new organizations called health and wellbeing boards bringing together local councillors with local clinicians to decide how health services will be provided. It will also give greater power to the public because they vote for the local councillors who are part of the decision-making process.

SELF CHECK 2.3

Why is it important for GPs to take over commissioning services for their patients?

2.4 **Clinical governance**

There are a number of definitions of **clinical governance**. One of the most frequently stated is: the framework through which NHS organizations are accountable for continuously improving the quality of their services and safeguarding high standards of care by creating an environment in which clinical excellence will flourish. This definition comes back to Bevan's view that services need to be constantly changing to meet patients' needs. It also enshrines another NHS philosophy: that the best possible care/treatment should be provided from the resources available. In economic terms this would be described as value for money or appropriate use of financial resources. Clinical governance therefore encapsulates the spirit of the NHS that states that high-quality care is available to all on demand, regardless of social status or wealth. So although the term clinical governance may be relatively new terminology (it has been around for just over a decade) it is a concept that has been present since the NHS was formed.

It should be clear from this definition that clinical governance affects every NHS organization and NHS employee, and can be seen in the structures of the organizations that have been described in this chapter. It should also be obvious that clinical governance has to underpin how professionals go about providing their care to patients.

Clinical governance is promoted as a mechanism to demonstrate quality to patients and the general public, provide confidence in the health care system, and demonstrate a minimum standard of uniformity in care across a wide geographical area. This is needed as high-profile cases of poor performance can easily damage the NHS's reputation. The better the clinical governance within an organization the lower the risk of such poor performance going unnoticed and unaddressed.

> **KEY POINT**
>
> Clinical governance is a mechanism to demonstrate quality in health care. By setting a minimum standard of uniformity in care across a wide geographical area patients and the general public can feel reassured.

What are the fundamental elements that make up clinical governance?

The definition of clinical governance refers to a framework for ensuring quality. This system will in fact be a set of policies and procedures that covers a range of topics. It is accepted that the framework should cover seven key areas, and these are sometimes described as the 'seven pillars of clinical governance' (Figure 2.2 and Table 2.1).

The concept of clinical governance was built upon by the Care Quality Commission in England. It is their role to determine whether care providers are complying with the essential standards of quality and safety. These standards specify what patients can expect from healthcare providers. The Commission has a range of powers it can use if it finds an organization falls short of the standards.

How does clinical governance work within pharmacy?

In community pharmacy, clinical governance is an essential service within the pharmacy contract. That means that every pharmacy has to provide the service.

FIGURE 2.2 Diagrammatic representation of the seven pillars of clinical governance. All seven key areas must be in place in order to have good clinical governance and the absence of one significantly weakens the overall standard.

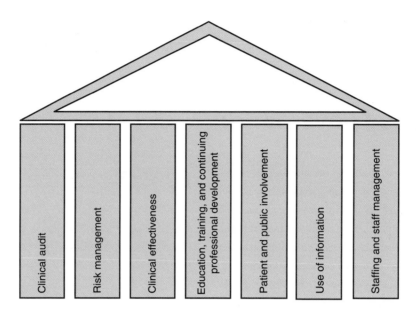

TABLE 2.1 The seven pillars of clinical governance

Pillar	Description
Clinical audit	This is a process by which health professionals can review and assess their current practice to see how it compares with current standards. Modifications can be made to improve the service, which can also be reviewed at a later date to ensure that real improvements have been obtained.
Risk management	It is impossible to completely eliminate the risk of patient or staff harm or injury but good systems can significantly reduce risks. This pillar is about having systems to monitor risk and initiate changes to address potential problems. It is particularly about learning from mistakes and creating a culture where preventing future occurrences is more important than blaming individuals for mistakes or errors. Recording and reporting incidents is an important element of this system.
Clinical effectiveness	This pillar is the epitome of clinical governance. Health care professionals need to keep up to date with changes in best practice and with the latest evidence on the best forms of treatment and care. If this is done all patients will receive the best quality of care available at that time in a consistent way.
Education, training, and continuing professional development	This is seen as the key to minimizing poor performance within individuals or within a team or organization. Health care professionals are expected to continue to expand their knowledge and understanding throughout their career. It is through this process that the previous pillar of clinical effectiveness can be achieved. Systems and processes need to be in place to support staff in complying with this requirement and give them the opportunity to strive for excellence.
Patient and public involvement	This is the critical pillar within clinical governance. It is vital that the NHS remains patient-centred and so collecting information from patients and carers on their experience of the NHS is a fundamental requirement. It is their perception of quality that is the most important and consequently good patient engagement allows services to develop in an effective manner.
Use of information	The use of data or information obtained on comparable services and the use of national or local standards allows services to be compared or benchmarked against others. Identifying poor performance against a particular standard can be used as a driver for change and lead to the creation of improved systems and procedures. If this comparison work were not undertaken it would be easy to assume that current performance was better than it really was.
Staffing and staff management	This is about the concept of creating an environment where excellence can flourish. It covers the entire process of employing staff, providing appraisals and training, and setting the organizational culture, as well as implementing systems to manage poor performance and non-compliance with policies and procedures such as disciplinary procedures.

The service specification covers each of the seven pillars. The key requirements for each pillar are described below.

Clinical audit

Each pharmacy in England must complete two clinical audits each year. One is a practice-based audit that is chosen by the pharmacy and the other is an audit that is chosen by the PCT. Both have an outcome that benefits patients.

Risk management

Pharmacies need to have a system for recording patient safety incidents, including all stages of the medication process and any near misses. A near miss in dispensing a prescription could be the dispensing of the wrong strength of a drug and would be classified as a near miss if the error was identified before the prescription medication was given to the patient. These incidents have to be reported to the NPSA or its successor organization. The analysis of incidents is required to ensure learning occurs so that future events can be minimized.

Pharmacies are also required to have standard operating procedures (SOPs) that cover the handling of a prescription from receipt to collection by a patient or their representative. The rationale behind SOPs is to ensure that there is a consistent standard of operation within the pharmacy that allows a uniform delivery of the service, regardless of who is working there on that day.

Patient safety notices and alerts concerning patient safety have to be acted upon within appropriate timescales and records kept of actions taken. An example of this could be the notification of pharmacies that a particular batch of aspirin 300 mg tablets issued by a supplier had accidently been packed in the boxes labelled as 75 mg tablets. The safety notice would ask the pharmacies to check their stock and remove from their shelves any stock from the batch identified in the safety notice.

Clinical effectiveness

Pharmacies must have protocols and SOPs to maintain the quality of self-care advice to patients. This is to ensure that there is a minimum standard that patients can expect and that all staff are following the same processes. There is a requirement for pharmacists to contribute to improving the clinical effectiveness of prescribing by following NICE guidance and evidence-based practice.

Education, training, and continuing professional development

Pharmacists have to demonstrate they are continuing their professional development (CPD); the pharmacy regulator (General Pharmaceutical Council or Pharmaceutical Society of Northern Ireland) can inspect the CPD records of pharmacists. In order to perform some additional roles pharmacists may be required to complete additional formal training. For example, pharmacists wishing to provide advice on safe handling and storage of medicines to care homes or wishing to perform medication use reviews are required to demonstrate that they have passed the appropriate assessments.

Patient and public involvement

Every pharmacy each year has to produce a patient satisfaction questionnaire and collect a number of responses from patients. The number of responses required is dependent on the volume of prescriptions dispensed by the pharmacy. The pharmacy has to analyse the results, take appropriate action, and publish the results.

The pharmacies have to produce a practice leaflet that outlines all the services available. It details the pharmacy opening hours and informs patients how they can complain or provide feedback on the services provided. Every pharmacy has to have a complaints system in place and use this to review the quality of its service provision.

Use of information

Pharmacies must possess appropriate up-to-date reference sources and are required to comply with information governance regulations and the data protection and confidentiality legislation. The Data Protection Act defines how patient data should be stored. Pharmacy staff should not divulge patient-sensitive information, such as the patient's age or medical treatment history, unless in accordance with circumstances identified within the Act.

Staffing and staff management

All staff must have appropriate training for their roles and should undergo appropriate induction training. Development needs of staff have to be identified and supported.

It is not just through the application of the clinical governance service that pharmacy adopted clinical governance as the mechanism to improve quality. Many new roles provided by pharmacists have qual- ity monitoring and improvement built into them or the role is to provide support and advice to others on best practice. Pharmacists working in secondary care also comply with clinical governance requirements that cover the seven pillars.

> **SELF CHECK 2.4**
>
> Why is clinical governance important to pharmacists?

CHAPTER SUMMARY

➤ The creation of the NHS over 60 years ago radically changed health care in the UK. The community pharmacist's role changed to that of a supplier of medicines.

➤ In recent years the role of the pharmacist has changed again, with a greater focus on using the therapeutic and clinical skills of the pharmacist.

➤ The basic structure of the NHS is the same in the constituent parts of the UK although there are differences in the terminology used to describe the various components of the health care system.

➤ The structure of the NHS is constantly under review and will go through many changes during your career as a pharmacist. The NHS was founded under the principle of constantly adapting, improving, and moving forward driven by the desire to meet patients' expectations and provide high-quality services. Be prepared for change and challenges and meet them head on.

➤ The majority of NHS funding is channelled through primary care although a large proportion of this funding ends up in secondary care.

➤ Clinical governance is about ensuring high-quality services are in place. There are seven pillars which support clinical governance and all these pillars must be present to ensure quality is not compromised.

FURTHER READING

For further information regarding the arrangements for pharmaceutical services in the different parts of the UK please see the relevant website.

Scotland

The Scottish Government. NHS workforce. <http://www.scotland.gov.uk/Topics/Health/NHS-Workforce>.

Northern Ireland

Department of Health, Social Services and Public Safety. <http://www.dhsspsni.gov.uk/index/about_dept.htm>.

Wales

NHS Wales. <http://www.wales.nhs.uk>.

England

Department of Health. <http://www.dh.gov.uk>.

Legal and ethical matters

DAI JOHN

Pharmacists and pharmacy students must be fully aware of their legal and ethical responsibilities. Ignorance is generally no defence in law or in regulatory proceedings. As pharmacists may experience legal and/or ethical dilemmas in practice they should be able to apply their knowledge of law and ethics to their professional judgements. This chapter seeks to outline what we mean by law and ethics as well as the legal and regulatory systems in which pharmacists practise.

Learning objectives

Having read this chapter you are expected to be able to:

- ➤ Outline the sources of law and the legal systems in the UK.

- ➤ Describe the differences and similarities between civil and criminal law.

- ➤ Outline the principles of health care ethics.

- ➤ Describe the different legal classes of medicines and explain the circumstances under which they may be supplied to the public.

- ➤ Describe how controlled drugs (substances controlled by the Misuse of Drugs Act) are categorized.

- ➤ Describe how the General Pharmaceutical Council (GPhC) aims to protect the health, safety, and well-being of people using pharmacy services.

- ➤ Explain the importance of fitness to practise issues.

3.1 The law and legal systems in the UK

Firstly, we will briefly cover the law and legal systems in the UK. We will introduce some important terms that will help you to understand the law in the context of the practice of pharmacy.

Background

'Great Britain' is a term used to denote England, Scotland, and Wales; that is, it excludes Northern Ireland. 'The UK' is a term that includes England, Scotland, Wales, and Northern Ireland. There are three major legal systems, each with their own legal rules, courts, and legal professions. These are based geographically: one in Northern Ireland, one in Scotland, and one covering England and Wales. 'English law' is the term often used to describe the law and legal system in England and Wales.

There are many similarities between the law and legal systems in the four home nations, but there are also some important differences. For example, the Human Medicines Regulations 2012 categorizes medicines for human use into three classes: POM (prescription-only medicines); P (pharmacy medicines); and GSL (general sale list medicines), and this classification applies across the UK. The General Pharmaceutical Council (GPhC) is the pharmacy regulator for England, Scotland, and Wales whereas the Pharmaceutical Society of Northern Ireland (PSNI) is the pharmacy regulator in Northern Ireland. Each of the four home countries determines its own regulations regarding charges that patients pay for NHS prescriptions.

> **KEY POINT**
>
> Medicines are classified by the Human Medicines Regulations 2012 as POM, P, or GSL.

The main types of law in the UK

Law can be classified as statute law or as common law. **Statute law** (or legislation) includes Acts of Parliament referred to as primary legislation. Regulations and orders, collectively referred to as statutory instruments (SIs) are made under the Acts and are referred to as secondary legislation. SIs usually contain a lot of detail. The Poisons Act 1972, the Misuse of Drugs Act 1971, and the Health Act 2006 are three examples of Acts that apply to the profession of pharmacy.

Common law has developed from the decisions of senior judges and is often referred to as **case law**. The decisions made by judges in the courts relate to the specific circumstances of a case where legislation does not exist or does not apply. An example relating to pharmacy is that pharmacists have a common-law duty of care to their patients and the public. The principles of common law have been developed as a result of cases heard over many years.

Public law or civil (private) law

Law can also be divided into public law and civil (or private) law. Public law involves the state or government. It includes criminal law, which determines behaviour forbidden by the state. Criminal law defines the boundaries of acceptable conduct. A person who contravenes criminal law is regarded as having committed an offence against society as a whole, which renders the offender liable to punishment by the state; for example, for theft. Another example of public law is administrative law, which controls how public bodies and individuals, including the NHS, community pharmacy contractors, and pharmacists, should operate. Examples of public law include the Misuse of Drugs Act 1971 and the Health Act 2006.

Civil law is concerned with disputes between individual persons or organizations regarding duties, rights, and obligations and, like public law, can be either statute law or common law. Examples of civil law include family law (adoption of children, divorce), property (land disputes, copyright infringements), law of contract (where there is a legally binding agreement between two parties), negligence, and defamation (libel, slander).

European Union law

The UK became a member of the European Union (EU) in 1973 and as a result needs to comply with EU law. The Court of Justice of the European Communities (often referred to as the European or the EU Court) can make regulations which are compulsory in all their elements and are directly applicable to all EU member states. This means that an individual state does not need to amend its national legislation. More commonly, the EU Court issues directives which are applicable to member states. Directives specify the objectives to be reached together and a time by which each state has to comply. It is up to individual states as to how the objectives are met; that is, how its law is amended so that it complies with the directive. In the UK, the most common means of incorporating directives into law is by means of secondary legislation as SIs. Where differences in law exist between EU and UK law, EU law is supreme.

The European Court of Human Rights is distinct from the European Court. The European Court of Human Rights enforces the European Convention on Human Rights. As a member state of the Council of Europe, the UK has agreed with the principles of the European Convention on Human Rights. The Human Rights Act 1998, which came into effect in October 2000, enables all the courts in the UK to protect the rights identified in this convention. Where an individual has exhausted their right to a hearing in a UK court they may, if that issue relates to their human rights, seek to have their case heard in the European Court of Human Rights.

3.2 Criminal law

A person who is alleged to have committed an offence (defendant) is prosecuted by the prosecution. If the defendant pleads guilty or is found to be guilty of the offence(s) then they are convicted and a criminal penalty is imposed. If they are found to be not guilty they are acquitted. A defendant who is accused of a number of offences could be found guilty of some offences and not guilty of others.

A decision to prosecute a defendant for an offence is usually made by the Crown Prosecution Service (England and Wales), by the Public Prosecution Service (Northern Ireland), or the Crown Office or by the Procurator Fiscal Service (Scotland). A decision to prosecute is based on evidence gathered by the police (and other agencies, including HM Revenue and Customs). The prosecution agency proceeds with a prosecution if it believes there is enough evidence to provide a reasonable prospect of obtaining a conviction and also if it is in the **public interest** to prosecute. For example, for a one-off very minor offence the individual may not be prosecuted.

The Medicines and Healthcare products Regulatory Agency (MHRA) may bring criminal prosecutions under certain circumstances such as unlawful manufacture, supply, or promotion of medicines. The MHRA is a government agency with responsibility for ensuring medicines and medical devices work and are acceptably safe. The MHRA has responsibility for enforcing medicines legislation in England, and does so in Scotland and Wales on behalf of the Scottish Parliament and Welsh Assembly, respectively. Department of Health lawyers (as opposed to the Crown Prosecution Service) usually conduct prosecutions. The MHRA works closely with the Department of Health, Social Services and Public Safety (DHSSPS) in Northern Ireland. The pharmacy regulator, the GPhC, can also prosecute a defendant for certain types of provision of medicines offences.

> **KEY POINT**
>
> Law can be divided into civil and criminal law and there are differences in the legal sanctions (remedies and punishments), systems, and terminology associated with each. There are similarities and differences between the legal systems in the four countries of the UK.

Burden and standard of proof in criminal cases

In simple terms, the **burden of proof** in criminal cases rests with the prosecution. The defendant bears no burden of proving anything and it is not his task to prove his innocence. That is, the prosecution must prove that the defendant is guilty.

The **standard of proof** required in a criminal trial by jury must convince the jury of the defendant's guilt. The prosecution proves its case if the jury, having considered all the evidence relevant to the charge, is sure that the defendant is guilty. Formerly, the standard of proof 'beyond all reasonable doubt' was used.

3.3 Civil law

A civil action is commenced by the **claimant** or aggrieved party. (The term 'plaintiff' was formerly used and you may see this term in some older textbooks and legal cases.) The claimant completes a claim form outlining details of the claim, such as the monetary value, and sends it to the appropriate court. The claimant sues (brings an action against) the defendant. (Note that the word defendant is the same word used in criminal law). The vast majority of civil cases are heard by one or more judges. Defamation is an example where trial by jury can be requested. Many civil cases are settled out of court to avoid legal and associated costs.

In civil law the burden of proof is on the claimant to prove his case. The standard of proof in civil proceedings is lower than in the criminal courts. In civil law the standard of proof required is on the **balance of probabilities**; that is, the claimant needs to prove it is more likely than not that the defendant has committed a civil wrong. (In civil law we do not use the term crime or criminal offence as we are not dealing with criminal law). In civil proceedings, if the defendant is found liable the judge will find in favour of the claimant and the judgement will determine what the defendant will need to do. For example, the defendant may be required to pay money (damages) to the claimant. Another civil remedy (judgement) such as an injunction may be issued, which requires, for example, the defendant to do something specific (or prevents them from doing something specific).

Negligence is a civil wrong. It requires the claimant to establish, for example, that:

1. the defendant owed a legal duty of care to the claimant;

2. the defendant was in breach of that duty of care; and

3. the claimant suffered loss or damage as a result of the defendant's breach of that duty of care.

Each one of these three elements must be proved by the claimant. The burden of proof is on the claimant and the standard which applies is on the balance of probabilities. The amount of damages awarded to the claimant is determined by the court after considering all the relevant evidence. The defendant is only liable for damages which are reasonably foreseeable as a result of the wrongful act or omission. Insurance companies provide professional indemnity insurance cover for pharmacists to cover them if an error is made and their patient suffers harm as a result of that error. One example of a negligent act by a community or hospital pharmacist is supplying the wrong drug to a patient who then suffers harm as a result of that error. Another example is where a medical doctor makes a mistake and prescribes too high a dose and the pharmacist dispenses it. If the patient suffered harm as a result of taking that dose then both the pharmacist and the doctor may be successfully sued in the civil courts.

SELF CHECK 3.1

Read the *British Medical Journal* article 'Writing a wrong' by Kenneth Mullan, which outlines two high-profile negligence cases, one decided in the High Court and the other in the Court of Appeal (Civil Division).

a. Who is the claimant (plaintiff) in the High Court case and who is the claimant (plaintiff) in the 1983 Court of Appeal case?

b. What is the standard of proof in civil cases such as these?

c. Is the burden of proof on the claimant (plaintiff) or on the defendant?

SELF CHECK 3.2

Give an example of a civil case that may be heard by a judge and jury.

3.4 **The UK courts**

Whether criminal or civil, common or statute law, the UK courts adhere to an accepted principle that any case is heard at the lowest possible tier of the court system. The court systems in England and Wales and in Northern Ireland are similar for both criminal and civil law.

If you look at Figure 3.1 you can see that the Supreme Court is the highest court in England and Wales and in Northern Ireland for both civil and criminal jurisdictions, and the magistrates' courts appear as the common lowest tier in these systems. Also, you can see that the county courts do not deal with criminal cases.

Comparing Figure 3.1 with Figure 3.2 (showing the structure of the Scottish courts), we can see that there a number of differences between English and Scottish courts. For example, the Justice of the Peace Courts are the lowest tier of criminal courts in Scotland. The Supreme Court has the highest civil jurisdiction in Scotland (as it has in England and Wales and in Northern Ireland) but it is the High Court of the Justiciary that is the supreme criminal court in Scotland. The Sheriff Courts serve both criminal and civil functions in Scotland.

Please check with your lecturers to see with which legal systems/courts you need to be familiar.

FIGURE 3.1   Court structure in England and Wales and in Northern Ireland (simplified)

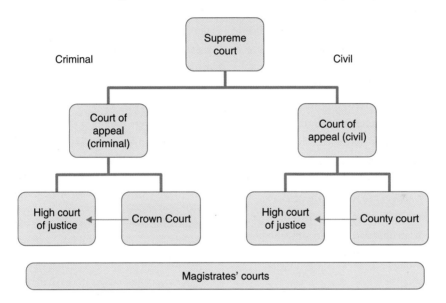

FIGURE 3.2   Court structure in Scotland (simplified)

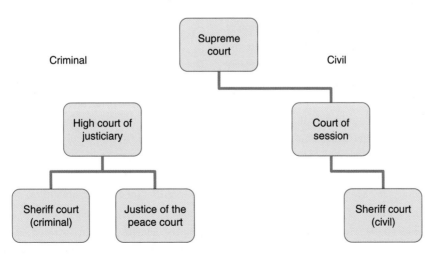

3.5 Courts in England and Wales and in Northern Ireland that deal with criminal cases

Magistrates' courts

Cases in the magistrates' courts are heard by a legally qualified magistrates' courts district judge or deputy district judge. In England and Wales (but not Northern Ireland) cases may also be heard by a panel of three lay magistrates (who are not legally qualified), and in such circumstances a legal adviser is available to the panel at all times. In criminal cases a magistrates' court cannot impose sentences of imprisonment that exceed 12 months (6 months for a single offence in England and Wales).

If the defendant is tried and convicted in the magistrates' court there may still be committal proceedings to the Crown Court for sentencing when the magistrates consider their sentencing powers are inadequate. (A Crown Court can issue much higher penalties than a magistrates' court.) Defendants accused of an indictable offence must first appear in a magistrates' court for committal proceedings, where the prosecution must satisfy the court there is an adequate case against the person accused; if so, the trial is heard in the Crown Court.

Types of offences

Offences are categorized in one of three ways in relation to which court will hear a case against a defendant. **Indictable offences** are more serious crimes that are tried on **indictment** (a formal charge or accusation of a serious crime) in the Crown Court (in England and Wales) by a judge and jury. **Summary offences** are less serious and are tried in magistrates' courts. Offences **triable either way** are those that, under certain circumstances, are triable either summarily in a magistrates' court or on indictment in the Crown Court. Each charge (offence) on the indictment is referred to as a 'count'.

For example, medicines legislation states that the sale of a pharmacy medicine from a registered pharmacy in the absence of a pharmacist would be a criminal offence and is triable either way. The law states that this person would be liable to a fine on summary conviction or, on conviction on indictment,

to a fine, to imprisonment for a term not exceeding 2 years, or to both.

This means that if there were to be a prosecution against that individual and the case was heard in the Crown Court (on indictment) the defendant, if found guilty, could be fined or imprisoned for up to 2 years or both fined and imprisoned. If the case were heard in the magistrates' court (summary trial) then it would not be possible to imprison that pharmacist because the penalty in a summary trial is restricted to a fine. The law states what the maximum penalty is and a one-off sale of medicines from a pharmacy in the absence of a pharmacist is unlikely to result in prosecution, let alone imprisonment. However, repeated sales of large quantities of medicines where members of the public came to harm might result in a prison sentence. Each case is judged according to the individual circumstances of the case.

> **KEY POINT**
>
> Magistrates' courts hear and determine less serious criminal cases such as minor theft, criminal damage, public disorder, and motoring offences (summary offences and some triable either way). The vast majority of criminal cases are heard and resolved in the magistrates' courts.

Crown Court

The Crown Court deals with crimes that are not classed as minor. All serious crimes such as murder, drug trafficking, and serious sexual offences are heard in the Crown Court. Cases in the Crown Court are heard in front of a judge and a 12-person jury (except terrorism cases in Northern Ireland, where there is no jury). The jury can be unanimous in its verdict (of guilty or not guilty) or the judge may accept a majority verdict of 11–1 or 10–2 (compare with the Sheriff Court in Scotland; see Section 3.6). The Crown Court also hears some appeals from magistrates' courts; for example, a defendant appealing against a sentence they believe is unduly severe. In Northern Ireland, both civil and criminal decisions of the magistrates' courts may be appealed to the county courts.

Court of Appeal

The Court of Appeal has a Criminal Division and Civil Division. Appeals against conviction or sentence from the Crown Court are heard in the Court of Appeal (Criminal Division).

Supreme Court

This is the highest criminal court in England and Wales and in Northern Ireland. Usually, five judges (but as many as nine) hear appeals from the Court of Appeal (Criminal Division).

3.6 The criminal courts in Scotland

Justice of the Peace Courts

A Justice of the Peace Court is a court where a Justice of the Peace (who is not legally qualified) sits with a legally qualified adviser, who provides advice on matters of law and procedure. There is a maximum term of imprisonment of 60 days. In Glasgow only, some courts are presided over by a legally qualified stipendiary magistrate and here the maximum term of imprisonment that can be imposed is 12 months.

Sheriff Courts: criminal jurisdiction

The Sheriff Courts deal with more serious criminal cases but not the most serious cases. There are two types of criminal trial, namely solemn (a sheriff, that is, a judge, sits with a 15-person jury) and summary trials (no jury). Following a 'solemn procedure' the court may impose a sentence of up to 5 years imprisonment. If a sheriff believes his or her sentencing powers are insufficient, the case may be referred to the High Court of Justiciary. Unlike criminal trials in the rest of the UK, in

Scotland a simple majority (8–7) is sufficient to establish whether or not the prosecution has proved its case. The maximum prison sentence that can be imposed in summary procedures is 12 months. Appeals against decisions in criminal cases can be made to the High Court of Justiciary. The Sheriff Courts also deal with many civil matters.

High Court of Justiciary

The High Court of Justiciary is the supreme criminal court for Scotland (other than for decisions involving matters of devolution). This court deals with the most serious crimes such as murder, drug trafficking, and serious sexual offences. Cases are tried by a judge and a 15-person jury. This court also has an appellate function, and when hearing appeals the trial is heard by at least two judges, without a jury. Appeals can be from criminal cases that have been heard in the Sheriff Court and also from criminal solemn trials heard for the first time in this court.

3.7 Criminal penalties (sentencing)

Legislation, for example, in an Act of Parliament, determines the maximum sentence for a particular criminal offence. If a defendant has pleaded guilty to, or has been found guilty of, more than one offence, in such circumstances the court may impose more than one penalty.

Discharges

Discharges are the most lenient sentence available to a criminal court. They are often given for minor offences such as minor theft or criminal damage where the court decides not to impose a punishment because the experience of appearing in court has been enough of a punishment itself. The defendant has pleaded guilty or has been found guilty by the court. An absolute discharge is where the offender is released without punishment and no further action is taken. A conditional discharge is where the offender is released without punishment on the condition that they must not commit any other offence within a specified time period (up to 3 years). If the offender is convicted of another offence within the specified period the court may impose a sentence for the original offence (for which the conditional discharge was imposed) as well as the new offence.

Fines

Fines are the most common type of sentence. The amount of fine is determined by the court and reflects the seriousness of the offence as well as the defendant's ability to pay. In certain circumstances, individuals who do not pay fines may be imprisoned.

Community orders

Community orders include community service, community supervision, and curfews. Other examples include alcohol or drug treatment orders where the defendant has an alcohol or drug problem. If an offender breaks the requirements of the community order they will be returned to court. In some cases offenders may be resentenced and could be imprisoned.

Custodial sentences

There is no capital punishment (death penalty) in the UK. Imprisonment is the most severe sentence available to the criminal courts. Prison (custodial) sentences are reserved for the most serious offences. They are used when the offence is so serious that neither a fine nor a community sentence can be justified for the offence and/or where the court considers imprisonment is necessary to protect the public. The length of the prison sentence depends on the maximum penalty for the crime, as outlined by statute, and on the circumstances of the offence and the offender. When there is more than one count on the indictment the court can impose sentences of imprisonment to run concurrently or consecutively.

The court may decide to suspend a prison sentence. This means the defendant is not imprisoned at that point. However, if the defendant is convicted of another crime within a specified period the court may impose a custodial sentence for the original offence as well as for the new offence(s). So, for example, a convicted defendant is given 6 months' imprisonment suspended for 2 years; this means that if there is a conviction for another offence within that 2-year period the defendant could go to prison for the original offence. The new offence would be dealt with by means of an appropriate penalty by the court, depending on the offence and facts of the case.

Examples of criminal convictions under the medicines legislation

Box 3.1 lists some examples of offences relating to medicinal products that have resulted in criminal convictions, some of which have involved a pharmacist. Very brief outlines of the offence for Case A to Case E are in normal font and the criminal penalty is in italic. Case F provides an example of a prosecution brought by the MHRA against a non-pharmacist for offences. We can see that failure to comply with a court order can result in a much more severe penalty; in this case a custodial sentence.

Ancillary orders

As well as imposing a sentence, a judge or magistrate may also impose additional orders known as ancillary orders. Examples of ancillary orders include antisocial behaviour orders (ASBOs), compensation orders, confiscation orders, disqualification from driving, travel restriction orders, and restraining orders.

BOX 3.1

Examples of criminal convictions under the medicines legislation

Case A: A pharmacist admitted (and was therefore convicted of) supplying ampoules of a prescription-only medicine (POM), in this case methadone, in the absence of a valid prescription.

- *The pharmacist dispensed a prescription that did not comply with all the requirements of the misuse of drugs legislation. They received a 2-year conditional discharge and had to pay court costs.*

Case B: A pharmacist was found guilty of selling medicinal products without a wholesale dealer's licence. The judge commented:

> The Medicines Act 1968 was passed to protect the public relating to the manufacture, sale and supply of medicines and any breaches of the Act should be treated seriously. As a pharmacist you are a professional person who has breached this trust and the sentence must reflect that position.

- *The pharmacist was fined and required to pay court costs.*

Case C: A non-pharmacist was convicted of four counts (four separate offences) of the sale of anabolic steroids (POMs) and one count of advertising POMs.

- *The individual was sentenced to 6 months' imprisonment on each count, to run concurrently.*

Case D: A private company advertised a POM (minoxidil for hair loss) to the public.

- *The company that owned the clinic was fined and ordered to pay costs.*

Case E: A non-pharmacist was convicted of 25 counts of importing POMs (anabolic steroids) into the UK without a product licence.

- *The individual was sentenced to 12 months' imprisonment on each count, to run concurrently, suspended for 2 years.*

Case F: On 14 January 2004 Peter Kaul (Mens Health Matters) was sentenced to 6 months' imprisonment, suspended for 2 years, for conspiracy and offences under the Medicines Act in relation to the illegal sale and supply of Viagra® (a POM).

- *On 14 May 2004 at Croydon Crown Court a confiscation order for £170 000 was made and the MHRA was awarded £15 000 costs.*

Kaul appeared in court several times regarding non-payment of the confiscation order. The matter was concluded on Tuesday 10 October 2006 at Marylebone Magistrates' Court. District Judge Arbuthnot stated:

> Mr Kaul has had over 2 years. No payment has been made. In my view he has not made any efforts to pay. He has had lots of opportunities including an asset he has failed to realize. He didn't sign the consent order, then he filed for bankruptcy, giving the same day's notice. I think I should issue the warrant for commitment.

- *Kaul was sent to prison for 3 years.*

Penalties where there has been no criminal court appearance

Not all criminal offences are dealt with by the courts. Police have a range of alternatives they can use to address minor (low-level) crimes. A caution is a formal warning given to an adult who has admitted an offence. If the person refuses the caution from the police then they may be prosecuted for the offence. A caution is not technically classed as a conviction but it can be taken into consideration by the courts if the person is convicted of another offence. A Criminal Records Bureau (CRB) check searches an individual's details against criminal records and other sources, including the

Police National Computer. The CRB check will either confirm that the individual does not have a criminal record or it will list any relevant convictions, cautions, or warnings and whether she or he has been prohibited from working with children or another vulnerable group. The police can also impose fixed penalties that may be relevant.

Fixed penalty notices (fines) can be issued by the police in a number of circumstances such as antisocial behaviour and certain minor traffic offences. They are not the same as criminal convictions but failure to pay the fine may result in a conviction and a penalty of higher fines or imprisonment.

Another example, although it is not a penalty, relates to provisions within the Mental Health Act 2007. This Act is unique in that it allows a person to be deprived of their liberty when they have neither committed a crime nor appeared before a court. Persons with a mental illness may be detained under the Act when detention is for the benefit of their own health, for their personal safety, or for the protection of others.

3.8 Pharmacists with criminal convictions

The notifiable occupations scheme

This scheme relates to professions and occupations which carry special trust or responsibility, and includes pharmacists. Police have a public interest duty to share with the GPhC or PSNI any convictions or other relevant information (for example, cautions) relating to pharmacists. So if you are cautioned or convicted of an offence the police will inform the regulator.

Rehabilitation of Offenders Act 1974

This Act generally allows individuals to start with a clean slate once sufficient time has elapsed since the conviction. After a certain time period, specific convictions are described as 'spent'. Once a conviction becomes spent individuals are not normally required to disclose it; for example, when applying for a job. However, this rule is subject to a number of important exceptions. Pharmacists are among a number of professionals who are *not* entitled to withhold information about previous convictions (even if they took place before registration as a pharmacist). Failure to disclose such convictions when applying for a job as a pharmacist or when seeking registration with the GPhC or PSNI can result in a fitness to practise investigation by the regulator.

3.9 Civil courts in England and Wales and in Northern Ireland

In Section 3.5 we looked at courts in England and Wales and in Northern Ireland that deal with criminal cases. In this section we turn our attention to civil courts.

Magistrates' courts

In addition to their role in criminal cases, magistrates' courts in England and Wales and in Northern Ireland also deal with civil matters such as family and domestic cases, applications for certain licences, and some relatively small debt cases.

County courts

The county courts in England and Wales and in Northern Ireland deal with most civil cases. Civil cases cover a wide range, such as personal injury, employment disputes, discrimination, and breaches of contract. Cases are heard by a judge without a jury. Decisions of the county courts may be appealed to the High Court. In Northern Ireland the county courts hear appeals from the magistrates' courts in both criminal and civil cases.

High Court

To give the courts their full names, the High Court of Justice in England and Wales and the High Court of Justice in Northern Ireland each consist of three divisions. These are namely the Chancery Division (cases involving financial matters such as trusts and mortgages, and companies), the Family Division (cases involving matrimony, custody of children), and the Queen's Bench Division, which deals with most other civil matters, such as medical negligence, defamation, and appeals from the inferior courts. The High Court deals with complex or important civil cases and hears appeals from the county courts. Cases are heard by a judge (almost always without a jury). Some decisions made by the High Court may be appealed to the Court of Appeal (Civil Division).

The Administrative Court of the Queen's Bench Division has a number of roles, including hearing appeals of pharmacists (and other professionals) whose right to practise has been removed or restricted by their regulatory body; for example, by the GPhC Fitness to Practise Committee.

Court of Appeal (Civil Division)

This court deals with appeals from the county courts, the High Court, and certain tribunals such as the Employment Appeals Tribunal in England and Wales and in Northern Ireland. Decisions of the Court of Appeal may under certain circumstances be appealed to the Supreme Court.

Supreme Court

This is the highest civil court in England and Wales, Northern Ireland, and Scotland. It hears appeals from the Court of Appeal (Civil Division) and in exceptional circumstances appeals from the High Court. It hears certain appeals from the Court of Session (Scotland). The Supreme Court replaced the House of Lords as the highest court in the UK in 2006.

3.10 Civil courts in Scotland

In Section 3.6 we looked at courts in Scotland that deal with criminal cases. In this section we turn our attention to civil courts.

Sheriff Courts: civil jurisdiction

The Sheriff Courts deal with many civil matters, such as discrimination, family matters, and various financial issues (for example, resolving financial disputes between individuals or organizations).

Court of Session and the Supreme Court

The Outer House hears cases at first instance (non-appeal cases) on a range of civil matters, including contract, negligence, and defamation. Cases are presided over by a judge (and, when appropriate, together with a civil jury). Decisions of the Outer House may be appealed to the Inner House of the Court of Session.

The Inner House mainly deals with appeals from the lower courts and from some tribunals and regulatory bodies, including the GPhC. Some decisions of the Inner House may be appealed to the Supreme Court.

3.11 Ethics

Ethics is the science of morals or moral philosophy. The principles that are accepted by a profession, such as pharmacy, as the basis of proper behaviour are the ethics of that profession. Ethics are usually codified into a formal set of rules, which are explicitly adopted by a profession to form a code of ethics governing the conduct of members of that profession. For example, the code of ethics for pharmacists in Great Britain is the GPhC's *Standards of Conduct, Ethics and Performance*. Similarly there is the GPhC's *Code of Conduct for Pharmacy Students*, as outlined in Chapter 1. Case Study 3.1 presents a situation covered by the GPhC standards.

 See Chapter 1 for more information on professional standards.

A breach of a principle within the GPhC standards may render the individual pharmacist subject to an investigation by the GPhC, which may result in a fitness to practise hearing, with the ultimate sanction being the removal of that individual's right to practise as a pharmacist.

Principles of health care ethics

More broadly in health care, four major biomedical ethical principles have been adopted internationally by health care professionals in relation to patients. Ethical decision-making usually involves at least one of these four principles, which are:

- *Autonomy*: respecting the choice/decision of an individual.
- *Non-maleficence*: avoiding harm.
- *Beneficence*: promoting well-being or doing good.
- *Justice*: similar individuals should normally have access to the same health care together with consideration of the fair distribution of limited resources.

CASE STUDY 3.1

You are a pharmacy student and you are undertaking a community pharmacy placement as part of your degree. While you are there, one of your university lecturers (Dr Patel) comes in with a prescription for an antidepressant. As this is the first time the lecturer (patient) has been prescribed this antidepressant the pharmacist talks to the patient about how to take the medicine, its side effects, and when she may expect to see an improvement in depression. The lecturer does not recognize you.

The following day in university you have a tutorial where you and five other students discuss your pharmacy placements. Your tutor asks you to describe an example of a situation where the pharmacist has counselled a patent on prescribed medication and you decide to talk about the lecturer and antidepressant. You mention Dr Patel's name.

REFLECTION QUESTION

Comment on this scenario. What did you do wrong? What might be the consequences?

Answer

You should not have disclosed this as it is confidential information. The GPhC *Standards of Conduct, Ethics and Performance* state: 'Respect and protect people's dignity and privacy. Take all reasonable steps to prevent accidental disclosure or unauthorized access to confidential information. Never disclose confidential information without consent unless required to do so by the law or in exceptional circumstances' (Principle 3.5). You may be subject to university fitness to practise procedures as you have divulged confidential information without consent. You could have discussed the facts in your tutorial, but you should not have mentioned the name of the person or other facts that could lead to her being identified.

Law, ethics, and morals

We have learnt that ethics can be considered as codes of conduct that relate to a group such as the pharmacy profession. Morality, however, refers to personal sets of beliefs about what is right and wrong. Morals not only come from within oneself but are also often learnt from cultural, religious, or other beliefs, from families, peers, society in general, or the media. Importantly, laws and morals are not opposites. The law has its basis in morals; in general the criminal law reflects the moral standards of the community.

Furthermore, while ethics can refer to a code of behaviour for a group, morals are more personal in nature. The difference between ethics and morality is highlighted when a person works as a member of a profession such as pharmacy or in an organization whose ethics are not in conformity with its morals. The GPhC guidance is contained in Standard 3.4 of the *Standards of Conduct, Ethics and Performance*. Standard 3.4 covers the provision of pharmacy services affected by religious and moral beliefs, and states that pharmacists must 'make sure that if your religious or moral beliefs prevent you from providing a service, you tell the relevant people or authorities and refer patients and the public to other providers'. This standard seeks to balance the need for patients to be able to access pharmaceutical services with respect for the religious or moral beliefs of pharmacy professionals. For example, if your beliefs prevent you from providing a pharmacy service such as emergency hormonal contraception, the guidance identifies what you should do prior to accepting employment, as well as how to deal with patients requesting such a service once you are employed.

> **SELF CHECK 3.3**
>
> What are the four main principles in health care ethics?

3.12 Outline of UK legislation relating to medicines for human use

The Medicines Act 1968 came into force in 1971. It is an enabling Act providing a system of licensing affecting the manufacture, importation, sale, and supply of medicinal products (or medicines) in the UK. The Human Medicines Regulations 2012 have replaced much of the Medicines Act 1968 and regulations made under it. The term medicines legislation is used to include the 1968 Act and the 2012 regulations. Enforcement of the requirements of the medicines legislation and offences are identified. The MHRA and a number of expert panels aim to ensure that, through legislation, medicines are of high quality and an appropriate balance between safety and effectiveness is achieved. The packaging, labels, and leaflets of medicinal products are required to meet the standards laid down in the Human Medicines Regulations 2012, as are prescribing information and requirements relating to the advertising and promotion of medicines. For further information on the MHRA see its website.

The definition of a 'medicinal product' for human use is found in the Human Medicines Regulations 2012 and is as follows:

1. Any substance or combination of substances presented as having properties for treating or preventing disease in human beings or

2. any substance or combination of substances that may be used by or administered to human beings with a view to:

   a. restoring, correcting, or modifying a physiological function by exerting a pharmacological, immunological, or metabolic action or

   b. making a medical diagnosis.

Medicines for human use are granted licences based on their safety, quality, and efficacy; these are the only three criteria on which the law controlling medicines for human use is founded (medicines for animal use are governed by the Veterinary Medicines Regulations). Pharmaceutical companies manufacture medicinal products in accordance with strict criteria. When quality is variable, safety and efficacy may become unpredictable. Quality of the final product depends on the source and purity of ingredients as well as the quantity and nature of impurities and excipients.

Uniformity of quality from one batch to another requires rigid adherence to specifications regarding ingredients and processes (including solvents and temperatures) during the manufacturing and formulation processes. Constant quality procedures at each stage of manufacture are demanded and records must be kept, which are subject to inspection by the MHRA. The proportions of different isomers, crystal forms of certain ingredients, and particle sizes, may affect the product. That is, quality must be built into the product (quality assurance) rather than be a single final test on the end product. After the product has been packaged and labelled, the medicine has to be stored and used appropriately, in accordance with its marketing authorization (MA). The packaging contains the MA number, which may be written as an equivalent PL number (the PL, or product licence, is a term formerly used to identify a licensed medicinal product and it applies to older medicines). Before being granted an MA the medicinal product is required to undergo a series of preclinical tests and clinical trials.

 See Chapter 11 in *Pharmaceutical Chemistry* within this series and Chapter 13 in *Pharmaceutics*, also in this series, for more information.

Before any medicinal product can be promoted it must have a licence (MA) and the company must produce a Summary of Product Characteristics (SPC). The SPC is produced for health professionals such as pharmacists and doctors, and contains information such as indications (uses), doses, cautions, storage, and special warnings.

 For further information on the drug development process, and the licensing of medicines and medicinal products, see Chapter 13 in *Pharmaceutics* within this series.

The Patient Information Leaflet (PIL) is included in the packaging that is supplied to the patient. The PIL contains less information than the SPC and is written in a style that is aimed at the patient. SPCs and PILs for medicines of some pharmaceutical companies can be found online in the searchable Electronic Medicines Compendium.

Legal classes of medicines for human use

The Human Medicines Regulations 2012 categorize medicines into three classes, namely general sale list (GSL) medicines, pharmacy (P) medicines and prescription-only medicines (POMs).

General sale list medicines (GSL)

GSL medicines can be sold to the public with reasonable safety from retail premises which can be closed to exclude the public; for example, supermarkets, shops, or fuel stations. Sales of GSL medicines from a market stall or car boot would be unlawful. GSL medicines can also be sold from pharmacies and may be supplied on prescription. Certain types of medicine cannot be GSL, irrespective of the ingredients. Consequently, none of the following are found as GSL medicines: parenteral products (injections); products for use wholly or mainly for irrigating wounds, the bladder, vagina, or rectum; or for use as anthelmintics (drugs to treat worm infestations).

Pharmacy medicines (P)

The container must contain a capital letter P in a box containing no other material: P. They can be sold to a member of the public from a registered pharmacy by, or under the supervision of, a pharmacist and they can be supplied on prescription. Some medicines are classed as pharmacy-only (PO) medicines (for example, Fybogel® 10 sachets). These medicines contain ingredients which are GSL but the licence only permits sale through a pharmacy.

Prescription-only medicines (POM)

A medicinal product is classified as a POM if it needs medical supervision to prevent a direct or indirect danger to human health, if it is widely and frequently misused and so presents a danger to health, if it is a new active substance, or if it is for parenteral administration. The label must contain POM, that is, the upper-case letters in a box with no other material. They may normally only be sold or supplied to a member of the public from a registered pharmacy by or under the supervision of a pharmacist in accordance with a valid prescription. There are many exemptions where the sale or supply to individuals other than members of the public is lawful; for example, to specific health professionals, to hospitals, and to universities for research or teaching.

Community pharmacists can also supply most (but not all) POMs to a patient in certain circumstances referred to as 'emergency supply', subject to a number of conditions being satisfied.

 See Chapter 5 for more information on prescribing and dispensing.

Legal class of medicines dependent on the pack size

Some medicines are GSL or P or POM depending on the 'pack size'; for example, the number of tablets within a container. Using paracetamol 500 mg non-effervescent tablets as an example, 16 is the maximum pack size available as a GSL medicine whereas 32 is the maximum pack size for sale as a P medicine. Packs containing more than 32 tablets are classed as a POM. There are also restrictions on the number of packs that

a community pharmacist can supply at any one time without prescription. Case Study 3.2 describes such a situation.

Legal class of medicines dependent on the strength

Some medicines are classed as GSL, P, or POM depending on their strength or concentration. For example, ibuprofen 400 mg tablets could be P or POM (but not GSL). Ibuprofen 600 mg tablets are POM.

SELF CHECK 3.4

Under what circumstances can a class P medicine lawfully be supplied to a member of the public without a prescription?

Misuse of Drugs Act 1971

The Misuse of Drugs Act 1971 is intended to control the movement and use of certain drugs. Its main aims are to make the following generally unlawful: manufacturing, supplying, or possessing controlled drugs (CDs); cultivating the cannabis plant; or using utensils or allowing others to use them in connection with the smoking of opium. There are exemptions; for example, the prescribing and dispensing for, and use by, patients where there is clinical need

CASE STUDY 3.2

You are working in a community pharmacy with a pharmacist. One day Mrs Thomas, a 64-year-old regular customer, asks for four packets of paracetamol 500 mg tablets (32 tablets per pack).

REFLECTION QUESTION

Would the pharmacist be able to sell Mrs Thomas the tablets?

to supply more than one packet.

for a week, the pharmacist may, under the circumstances, decide unable to obtain a prescription from her doctor for more tablets had run out of paracetamol prescribed by her doctor, and was elderly and had osteoarthritis of the knees, had difficulty walking,

The criminal law states that up to 100 paracetamol tablets can be sold as a P medicine. Therefore, the sale would be unlawful. Lawfully, a pharmacist could supply three packs of 32 tablets as the total is 96 tablets. Paracetamol is dangerous in overdose in that it can cause irreversible liver damage. In addition to considering the law the pharmacist has to consider the GPhC Standards of Conduct, Ethics and Performance first principle, which states: 'make patients your first concern'. For example, if the lady was depressed and wanted the tablets so she could take an overdose (96 tablets) then it is possible that she would end up with liver damage and may die. Clearly, the pharmacist should take care not to provide tablets to such a person even though it would be lawful. However, on the other hand, the same lady may be going on holiday for three weeks with her partner and three adult children, and it may be that she wishes to buy paracetamol for pain relief while they are away. The pharmacist may consider these circumstances as being appropriate to supply the three packs. If the lady was

Answer

or for research and teaching purposes. Where these exemptions are permitted there are a number of requirements. The government also restricts some CDs to research use only and can restrict professionals such as doctors or pharmacists from prescribing, dispensing, or possessing CDs in the course of their professional practice.

Class A, B, and C

The Misuse of Drugs Act 1971 classifies compounds into three categories according to their potential for harm; so the greater the potential for harm the greater the penalties in criminal courts. Drugs categorized as Class A have the greatest potential for harm and Class C have the least.

- *Class A* drugs include cocaine, ecstasy, diamorphine (heroin), lysergic acid diethylamide (LSD), and opium (raw, prepared, or medicinal). Also, any preparation containing a Class B when designed for administration by injection is Class A.

- *Class B* drugs include the following, unless they are designed for administration for injection: amphetamines, barbiturates, codeine, dihydrocodeine, and cannabis.

- *Class C* drugs include the benzodiazepines (such as temazepam and diazepam), anabolic steroids, and ketamine.

Penalties

Possession of a controlled drug and supply of a controlled drug are offences triable either way. The maximum penalty depends on the court in which the trial takes place and the class of drug.

 See Section 3.5 for more information on offences triable either way.

Using the England and Wales criminal courts as an example, Table 3.1 shows the maximum penalty (term of imprisonment) for a trial on indictment and a summary trial for each of the three classes using the offences of 'possession' and 'supply' of a controlled drug.

In Table 3.1 we can see that the maximum term of imprisonment for the Class A drug offences are higher than those for Class B or Class C. We can also see that the maximum penalty for a trial on indictment is greater than that available following a summary trial

TABLE 3.1 Examples of maximum penalties for possession and supply of Class A, B, and C drugs

Drug	Trial	Maximum prison sentence
Class A		
Possession	S	6 months
	I	7 years
Supply	S	6 months
	I	Life
Class B		
Possession	S	3 months
	I	5 years
Supply	S	6 months
	I	14 years
Class C		
Possession	S	3 months
	I	2 years
Supply	S	3 months
	I	14 years

I, Trial on indictment; S, Summary trial.

SELF CHECK 3.5

What is the maximum prison sentence available to a person convicted on indictment of supplying a Class B controlled drug?

for an equivalent offence under the Misuse of Drugs Act 1971.

Misuse of Drugs Regulations

Numerous regulations have been made under the Misuse of Drugs Act 1971 regarding the requirements that control the lawful possession, supply, record-keeping, storage, prescription requirements, and use of CDs; for example, when stored, prescribed, dispensed, or used as medicines. These regulations are of particular importance to pharmacists because a breach of the regulations renders the pharmacist subject to prosecution and a criminal conviction, even where the breach was not deliberate.

The regulations classify CDs into one of a number of schedules, with Schedule 1 having the most and Schedule 5 having the fewest controls associated with their lawful use.

 See Chapter 5 for more on prescribing and dispensing.

Schedule 1: (CD Lic POM)

A Home Office licence is required even to possess drugs in this schedule. It includes drugs that currently have no, or virtually no, therapeutic use, such as cannabis herb/resin, LSD, and ecstasy.

Schedule 2: (CD POM)

This includes amphetamines, diamorphine, methadone, and cocaine. There are particular requirements on storage and record-keeping as these are the most susceptible to misuse. Under the Human Medicines Regulations 2012 all would be classed as POMs.

Schedule 3: (CD No Register POM)

This includes buprenorphine, barbiturates, and temazepam and have less stringent requirements. All are classed as POMs.

Schedule 4, Part I: (CD Benz POM)

Contains most benzodiazepines (for example, diazepam). All are POMs.

Schedule 4, Part II: (CD Anab POM)

Contains anabolic steroids and growth hormones (for example, nandrolone, testosterone), which are all POMs.

Schedule 5: (CD Inv POM or CD Inv P)

These preparations contain certain CDs that are exempt from full controls; some are POM whereas others are P. Examples include codeine phosphate tablets (POM), codeine linctus (P), co-codamol 8:500 tablets (P), co-codamol 30:500 tablets (POM), pholcodine linctus (P) and Oramorph® oral solution 10 mg/5 ml (POM). Codeine injection is a Schedule 2 drug.

> **KEY POINT**
>
> Misuse of drugs legislation classifies medicines into five schedules with varying degrees of restrictions as to their use in practice.

> **SELF CHECK 3.6**
>
> Under the Misuse of Drugs Regulations, which schedules of drugs may a pharmacist lawfully possess in the course of his practise without the need of a licence from the Home Office?

3.13 Fitness to practise and the GPhC (Great Britain)

In addition to complying with criminal law, pharmacists and pharmacy technicians are expected to comply with standards set by the pharmacy regulator, the GPhC.

Some pharmacists are registered with both the PSNI and the GPhC and so would be subject to investigation by either organization. The GPhC's inspectors investigate complaints made against registered pharmacists, registered pharmacy technicians, and pharmacy owners. The complaints come from a variety of different sources including other registrants, employers, patients, members of the public, other health care professionals, primary care organizations, and other regulatory and enforcement authorities such as the police or the MHRA. Complaints could include reports of convictions, dispensing mistakes, or breaches of the principles contained in the GPhC's *Standards of Ethics, Conduct and Performance*. At the conclusion of an investigation the evidence is reviewed. Depending on the outcome of that review the complaint is referred to the Investigating Committee or the GPhC will write to the registrant outlining, with reasons, that there is to be no referral and sometimes offering advice.

 See Chapter 1 for more on the GPhC standards.

Investigating Committee

The Investigating Committee is a screening committee and meets in private. It considers all documents and relevant information, and any written explanations made by the registrant involved in the allegation. It does not hear oral evidence. It is required to consider all cases referred to it and decides whether or not an allegation should be referred to the Fitness to Practise (FtP) Committee.

It will refer a case to the FtP Committee where there is a real prospect that there will be a finding that the registrant's fitness to practise is currently impaired. If the Investigating Committee determines that the case does not need to be referred, it may:

- dismiss the case;
- give a warning to the registrant and decide that details of the warning should be recorded in the register;
- give advice to the registrant or any other person or organization involved in the investigation;
- agree undertakings with the registrant;
- decide that a criminal prosecution should be initiated.

Fitness to Practise Committee

The FtP Committee must act in the public interest when considering fitness to practise issues; that is, its decisions need to:

- protect members of the public;
- maintain public confidence in the profession;
- declare and uphold proper standards of conduct and behaviour.

The FtP Committee exercises discretion in a way that is fair and reasonable, weighs the interests of practitioners against the public interest, and considers the range of sanctions available to it before deciding on which to impose. The FtP Committee must consider its indicative sanctions guidance. If the FtP Committee finds that a registrant's fitness to practise is impaired it may impose one of the following sanctions:

1. Issue a warning.
2. Issue advice to anybody appropriate (for example, to the GPhC, to an employer, or to the profession).
3. Impose conditions for up to 3 years (for example, the registrant cannot work as a sole pharmacist).
4. Suspend the registrant from the register (meaning they are unable to practise for up to 12 months).
5. Directly remove the name of the registrant from the register—the ultimate sanction.

Individuals may only appeal through the courts against sanctions 1, 2, and 3. Registrants residing in England and Wales appeal to the High Court (Administrative Court of the Queen's Bench Division) or, if resident in Scotland, to the Court of Session.

SELF CHECK 3.7

Which GPhC committee/s has/have the power to remove a pharmacist's name from the register?

The registrant is entitled (under common law) to:

- an unbiased hearing;
- a right to be present and to be represented; and
- a right to be informed of the reasons for the decision.

Also, article 6(1) of the European Convention on Human Rights entitles the registrant to:

- a fair and public hearing;
- within a reasonable time; and
- by an independent and impartial tribunal established by law (in this case the GPhC's FtP Committee).

The underlying principle of the FtP Committee is to determine whether or not a registrant's fitness to practise is currently impaired and, if so, whether or not a sanction should be imposed. It receives evidence, including oral evidence, and usually sits in public (there are some circumstances where certain evidence is heard in private, such as matters relating to personal health issues or evidence relating to children). The burden of proof is on the GPhC to prove the facts of the case against a registrant, and the civil standard of proof of the balance of probabilities applies. The decision is made in public and reasons for the decision are given. The written decisions (referred to as determinations) are uploaded onto the GPhC website and are publicly available.

 See Section 3.3 'Civil law' for information on the burden of proof and balance of probabilities.

Impairment of fitness to practise

A registrant's fitness to practise may be impaired for one or more of a number of reasons, including misconduct, poor performance, and ill health. Section 51 of The Pharmacy Order 2010 contains the legal definition, which is provided in Box 3.2.

53

BOX 3.2

Definition of impaired fitness to practise (extract from the Pharmacy Order 2010)

Section 51:

1. A person's fitness to practise is to be regarded as 'impaired' for the purposes of this Order only by reason of:

   a. misconduct;

   b. deficient professional performance (which includes competence);

   c. adverse physical or mental health which impairs their ability to practise safely and effectively or which otherwise impairs their ability to carry out the duties of a pharmacist or a pharmacy technician in a safe and effective manner;

   d. failure to comply with a reasonable requirement imposed by an individual assessor or an assessment team in connection with carrying out a professional performance assessment;

   e. a conviction in the British Islands for a criminal offence;

   f. a conviction elsewhere than in the British Islands for an offence which, if committed in England, Wales or Scotland, would constitute a criminal offence;

   g. an order under section 246(2) or (3) of the Criminal Procedure (Scotland) Act 1995 discharging the person absolutely (admonition and absolute discharge);

   h. having accepted a conditional offer under section 302 of the Criminal Procedure (Scotland) Act 1995 (fixed penalty: conditional offer by procurator fiscal);

   i. having agreed to pay a penalty under section 115A of the Social Security Administration Act 1992 (penalty as alternative to prosecution);

   j. a police caution in the British Islands;

   k. having agreed to be bound over to keep the peace by a magistrates' court in England or Wales;

   l. a determination made by a regulatory body in the UK responsible under any enactment for the regulation of a health or social care profession to the effect that the person's fitness to practise as a member of a profession regulated by that body is impaired, or a determination by a regulatory body elsewhere to the same effect;

   m. the Independent Barring Board including the person in a barred list (within the meaning of the Safeguarding Vulnerable Groups Act 2006 or the Safeguarding Vulnerable Groups (Northern Ireland) Order 2007; or

   n. the Scottish Ministers including the person in the children's list or the adults' list within the meaning of the Protection of Vulnerable Groups (Scotland) Act 2007.

2. The demonstration towards a patient or customer, or a prospective patient or customer, by a pharmacist or pharmacy technician of attitudes or behaviour from which that person can reasonably expect to be protected may be treated as misconduct for the purposes of paragraph (1)(a).

3. References in this article to a conviction include a conviction by court martial.

4. A person's fitness to practise may be regarded as impaired because of matters arising:

   a. outside Great Britain; and

   b. at any time.

Applying for restoration to the register

Registrants whose names have been removed from the register may apply for restoration to the register after a period of no less than 5 years. The FtP Committee will consider the application and may allow or refuse restoration. The burden of proof is on the applicant to prove that they are entitled to be registered and the civil standard applies (balance of probabilities). If the FtP Committee allows registration it may impose conditions on that individual for up to 3 years. If restoration is refused, the individual has a right of appeal to the High Court (or Court of Session in Scotland).

GPhC Appeals Committee

A person (such as a pre-registration pharmacist) may be refused initial registration owing to impaired fitness to practise; for example, on health grounds, character, and/or for a previous conviction. The refusal can occur after the individual has graduated and otherwise successfully completed their pre-registration year. The applicant may in certain circumstances appeal against the decision not to register them and they may do so via the GPhC Appeals Committee. The Appeals Committee receives evidence, including oral evidence, and the decisions available include dismissal of the appeal (meaning the individual is not permitted to register as a pharmacist) or to allow the appeal and thereby permit registration with the GPhC. The burden of proof is on the applicant and the standard of proof is the civil standard, on the balance of probabilities. Appeals against a decision of the Appeals Committee can be made to the county court (or Sheriff's Court if the individual resides in Scotland).

KEY POINT

The GPhC is the regulator for pharmacy. It sets standards for pharmacists and pharmacy technicians (and for pharmacy premises). Falling short of one or more of these standards may result in proceedings that impose restrictions on an individual's practice. Pharmacists need to be aware of the laws and ethical standards that apply to their practice and as they experience legal and/or ethical dilemmas in practice. They should be able to apply the knowledge of law and ethics to their professional judgements.

SELF CHECK 3.8

If the GPhC Fitness to Practise Committee removes a pharmacist's name from the register, to which court may that pharmacist appeal if they reside (a) in England or Wales and (b) if they reside in Scotland?

3.14 Veterinary medicines

The Veterinary Medicinal Products Directive 2001/82/EC (as amended) describes the controls on the manufacture, authorization, marketing, distribution, and postmarketing surveillance of veterinary medicines. The regulations are updated approximately annually to ensure that they are up to date and fit for purpose. Medicines for animal use are assigned to one of five categories, some of which can be supplied by a pharmacist. For further information on veterinary medicines see the Department for the Environment, Food and Rural Affairs' Veterinary Medicinal Products Directive website.

CHAPTER SUMMARY

➤ An understanding of law, legal systems, ethics, and professional judgement is vital to the role of pharmacists.

➤ This chapter introduced a legal and ethical context in preparation for application of legal and ethical principles in later years of study and in practice.

➤ The sources of law and the legal systems in the UK have been outlined. The major differences and similarities between civil and criminal law and the principles of health care ethics have been provided.

➤ In terms of medicines and drugs, the chapter has described the three legal classes of medicines (POM, P, and GSL) and described how controlled drugs are categorized.

➤ The reader has also been made aware of how the General Pharmaceutical Council (the pharmacy regulator) aims to protect the health, safety, and well-being of people using pharmacy services, including the importance of fitness to practise issues.

FURTHER READING

Wingfield J. (Ed.) *Dale and Appelbe's Pharmacy and Medicines Law.* 10th edn. Pharmaceutical Press, 2013.

> This textbook provides an outline of the law that affects the practice of pharmacy in Great Britain. It provides considerable detail on the law relating to medicines for human and animal use, including controlled drugs and other laws relating to pharmacy.

Royal Pharmaceutical Society. *Medicines, Ethics and Practice. The Professional Guide for Pharmacists.* Pharmaceutical Press. Published annually.

> This guide has been developed as an underpinning document to help pharmacists with legal, ethical, and professional issues that commonly arise in practice. It has been written to support pharmacists in their day-to-day practice and embeds professional judgement and professionalism in the decision-making process.

4

Public health

JOSEPH BUSH

Public health is as old as civilization itself and is focused on improving the health of populations. For as long as the pharmacy profession has existed, pharmacists have contributed to improving the health of the population. The under-utilization of community pharmacy as a public health resource has been acknowledged and attempts have been made to address this via the policy process (including the new pharmacy contract). Pharmacy's contribution to public health is attracting renewed attention as health services are reconfigured to meet the needs of the population. All schools of pharmacy will address the topics in this chapter but many may not label these as 'public health'. An awareness of the breadth of public health topics and an understanding of the pharmacist's contribution to these is necessary if students are to make a full contribution to health care.

Learning objectives

Having read this chapter you are expected to be able to:

➤ Outline how health is commonly defined.

➤ Understand the many and varied determinants of the health status of individuals.

➤ Define public health and describe the public health approach.

➤ Describe the historical development of the public health movement with reference to key figures and policies.

➤ Describe contemporary public health practice and how it is influenced by government policy.

➤ Outline pharmacy's historical contribution to public health and how the pharmacy policy agenda has developed the public health function of pharmacists.

➤ Discuss the current nature of pharmacy's public health function.

➤ Describe how health is measured.

4.1 What is health?

The answer to the question posed in the heading of this section may appear—at first sight—to be very simple to answer. However, 'health' is surprisingly difficult to define. To provide but one confounding factor, an individual's age may alter their perception of health or what is 'healthy'. For example, a neonate may be considered healthy if he/she is free from illness and developing normally, an adolescent or young adult may consider themselves healthy if they are free from physical and mental illness, whereas an elderly person may consider themselves healthy when their arthritis and bronchitis are not 'playing up'.

One common thread throughout all the above examples is the presence, management, or absence of illness, most commonly conceptualized in the form of 'disease'. However, in a similar fashion to discussions around a definition of health, diseases share no single, common characteristic. The *Concise Oxford English Dictionary* definition of disease is 'a disorder of structure or function in a human, animal, or plant, especially one that produces specific symptoms or that affects a specific part.' Employing this definition, it is possible to perceive any factor that produces symptoms within an organism as a 'disease'. A 1979 study published in the *British Medical Journal* found that around a quarter of general practitioners (GPs) considered starvation to be a disease.

One thing we can say with confidence is that although disease and health may be treated as distinct entities neither can be said to exist without being associated with an organism. We can then describe the organism as being healthy or having a disease. This is not to say that a person cannot have a disease and still be healthy, but pharmacists (and all medical scientists) commonly view health in this manner—a person without an ailment is considered to be healthy.

This particular conceptualization of health is synonymous with the 'biomedical model of health'. This model of health dates back to at least the seventeenth century and was influenced by the work of the philosopher René Descartes. The biomedical model takes a mechanistic view of the body. Essentially the body is a machine; illness is its malfunctioning. In this context health is the absence of illness.

 See Chapter 7 for more in-depth coverage of models of health.

The biomedical model remained the dominant model until at least the middle of the twentieth century, when medicine was subjected to vehement criticism from the likes of Thomas McKeown. Such work established the idea of a 'social' model of health on the professional mind map.

 See Section 4.4 for more details of Thomas McKeown's work.

The social model conceives health as an interaction between body, mind, and environment. Figure 4.1 highlights how health is influenced by a multitude of different determinants, ranging from society-level factors through to individual hereditary factors.

The determinants of health can be split into 'upstream', 'midstream' and 'downstream'. Upstream factors are those under national control and include social, physical, economic, and environmental factors such as education, employment, income, and housing. These appear towards the outside of Dahlgren and Whitehead's model. Midstream factors are intermediate level factors that affect defined populations such as local communities, schools, or universities, and include local availability of healthy choices such as diet, facilities for exercise, and safe neighbourhoods. Downstream factors include individual lifestyle factors (such as smoking, alcohol intake, and diet) and demographic and hereditary factors that an individual has no influence over. These appear towards the inside of the model.

SELF CHECK 4.1

What are upstream and downstream determinants of health?

Approaches and interventions that tackle upstream factors are likely to result in the greatest impact on population-wide differentials. However, such society-level changes are the most difficult to bring about as well as being the most politically sensitive. Action that is targeted towards defined populations such as local communities are midstream interventions. Policies that address downstream factors, while still important, probably only serve to improve individual health.

 See Section 4.8 for more discussion around population-based health.

This section has highlighted the differences in how we perceive health and the difficulty in defining health concisely. Arguably the most widely used and quoted definition of health is from the constitution of the World Health Organization (WHO).

FIGURE 4.1   The determinants of health.
Source: Dahlgren G, Whitehead M. (1991). *Policies and Strategies to promote social equity in health*. Stockholm, Sweden: Institute for Futures Studies.

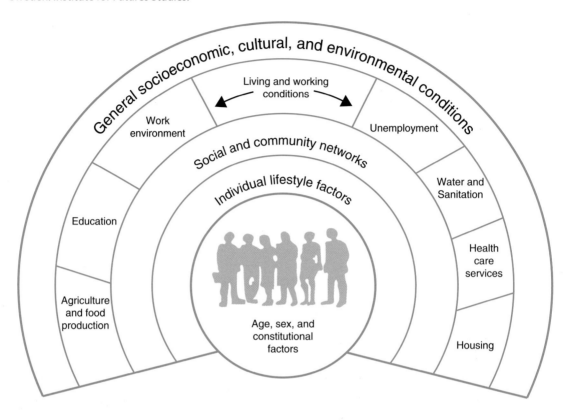

KEY POINT

The WHO defines health as 'a state of complete physical, mental and social well-being and not merely the absence of disease or infirmity'.

It is this definition, with an emphasis on an overarching sense of well-being, not just on the absence of disease, which we should refer to in our everyday studies and practice in pharmacy.

4.2 Measuring health: epidemiology

Epidemiology is an essential part of public health research that informs policy development and evidence-based medicine. Epidemiology is defined (Last, 1988) as 'the study of the distribution and determinants of health-related states or events in specified populations and the application of this study to the control of health problems'. Epidemiologists measure disease frequency in populations. They study sick and well people to determine the crucial differences between those who get ill and those who are spared.

An epidemic is defined as 'the occurrence in a community or region of cases of an illness, specific health-related behaviour, or other health-related events clearly in excess of normal expectancy'. Epidemics are contrasted with diseases that are endemic, which are constantly present in a given area, usually at low levels (see Figure 4.2). The term 'pandemic' refers to an epidemic spread over a wide geographic area (such as a continent or the whole world) and affecting a large proportion of the population.

FIGURE 4.2 Epidemic versus endemic disease

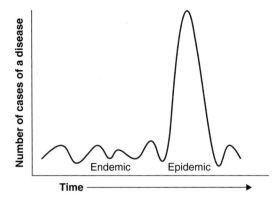

KEY POINT

An epidemic is an unexpected excess of cases of an illness, health-related event, or health-related behaviour within a specific population.

There is no single standard measure of the health status of populations, although life expectancy is commonly used as a proxy measure. Life expectancy is the number of years an individual can expect to live at a certain point in their life course, most usually at the point of their birth. Healthy life expectancy is a related statistic which estimates how many years an individual might expect to live in good health (before the development of a life-limiting illness, for example). When considering the health status of populations epidemiologists use rates; for example, the number of events that occur in a given population, where the number of events is the number of people to whom something happened (for example, those who died or contracted a disease) and the population is the population at risk (the total number of people to whom that event could happen). Some of the rates more commonly used in epidemiology are incidence, prevalence, and mortality.

Incidence

Incidence is the rate at which *new* cases of a condition occur in a population within a specified time period. For example, the incidence of tuberculosis in the UK in 2009 was 12 per 100 000 population per year. Once a person has been classified as a 'case' (for example, when they have been diagnosed with tuberculosis)

their status is defined and they cannot become a new case. Incidence refers only to new cases, not total cases.

Prevalence

Prevalence is the proportion of a population that are *new and old* cases at a given time. It can be calculated using the following formula:

$$prevalence = \frac{a}{a+b}$$

Where a = the number of individuals in the population with the disease at a given time and b = the number of individuals in the population without the disease at a given time.

Prevalence can be measured at a particular point in time (point prevalence) or over a specified period of time such as 1 year (period prevalence). The prevalence of tuberculosis in the UK in 2009 (point prevalence measured in the middle of the calendar year) was 15 per 100 000 population.

Mortality rates

Mortality rates are a measure of the number of deaths in a population during a specific period. These 'crude' mortality rates are rarely useful owing to significant variations within populations. More specific mortality rates include:

- *Maternal mortality rate*: the number of maternal deaths due to childbearing per 100 000 live births.
- *Perinatal mortality rate*: the sum of neonatal deaths and fetal deaths (stillbirths) per 1000 births.
- *Infant mortality rate*: the number of deaths of children less than 1 year old per 1000 live births.
- *Child mortality rate*: the number of deaths of children less than 5 years old per 1000 live births.
- *Standardized mortality rates*: as crude rates are often inappropriate, mortality rates can be standardized to take account of differences between populations, such as age. The age-standardized mortality rate for a given population (for example, the population of Birmingham) is the number of deaths, usually expressed per 100 000, that would occur in that population if it had the same age structure as a defined 'standard' population (for example, the population of the UK) and the age-specific rates of the population being studied applied.

4.3 What is public health?

In its simplest form, public health refers to the health of a population, the life expectancy of its members, and the extent to which they are free from disease. It implies a focus on the health states of populations rather than individuals. Public health has traditionally had a strong collective focus, placing an emphasis on collective action (for example, by government) to improve health.

The Faculty of Public Health (FPH) is the standard-setting body for specialists in public health in the UK. Most work within public health principally falls within the FPH's three key domains of public health practice: health improvement, improving services, and health protection, which you can see in Table 4.1.

Concise definitions of public health within the UK vary, but the majority are based on the definition of public health devised by Sir Donald Acheson in his 1988 report *Public Health in England*: 'The science and art of preventing disease, prolonging life and promoting, protecting and improving health through organized efforts of society.'

SELF CHECK 4.2

Within a population, who has responsibility for health improvement?

4.4 Public health through the ages

It can be argued that public health is as old as civilization itself. For example, there is evidence to suggest that the Ancient Greeks drained marshland in an effort to prevent malaria (although they erroneously believed malaria to be caused by drinking swamp water rather than it being transmitted by the mosquitoes that thrived in such environments). In the UK, the origins of public health are widely perceived to be rooted in the nineteenth century.

'Old' public health: sanitary reform in the UK

The rapid industrialization of Britain in the early nineteenth century led to an influx of people to the newly industrialized towns and cities. For example, the population of Birmingham increased from around 85 000 in 1811 to over 500 000 in 1901. Towns and cities were often unable to cope with such mass migration and the problems brought in its wake.

The majority of these economic migrants were confined to slums. Houses were small, overcrowded, and poorly ventilated, with shared toilet facilities. Open

sewers would run down the courses of the narrow streets. In such conditions, epidemics of infectious diseases were common. During the middle of the

TABLE 4.1 The Faculty of Public Health's three key domains of public health practice

Health improvement	Improving services	Health protection
Inequalities	Clinical effectiveness	Infectious diseases
Education	Efficiency	Chemicals and poisons
Housing	Service planning	Radiation
Employment	Audit and evaluation	Emergency response
Family/community	Clinical governance	Environmental health hazards
Lifestyles	Equity	
Surveillance and monitoring of specific disease and risk factors		

nineteenth century, infectious disease was responsible for a third of all deaths in England and Wales and life expectancy for labouring men in Liverpool fell to just 15 years.

The dominant belief at the time was that disease was caused by *miasma*: foul smells. The facts documented by reformers of the age, and the belief that disease was caused by filthy living conditions and a poor physical environment, highlighted the need for sanitary reform.

Foremost among the sanitary reformers of the Victorian age was Sir Edwin Chadwick. In 1842 Chadwick produced his *Report on the Sanitary Condition of the Labouring Population of Great Britain*, which, among other things, outlined the plight of the urban poor, detailed the wide discrepancies in life expectancy between the labouring and professional classes, and suggested that insanitary conditions were responsible for the increased death rates among the working classes.

Chadwick became the champion of the 'sanitary idea' of public health through public works, based on the principle that it is a public duty to prevent infectious disease by providing water that is pure and sewers that will safely remove what is dangerous. His commitment to sanitary reform was not wholly based on an altruistic desire to improve the lot of the poor. Chadwick, who was Secretary of the Poor Law Commission (the commission responsible for the system of relief for those in poverty), believed that good health equalled good economics: improved sanitation would further reduce the burden on local ratepayers of relief for the poor by ensuring that male breadwinners did not succumb to acute infectious diseases.

Chadwick's work led to the Public Health Act of 1848, by which, for the first time, the British government charged itself with a measure of responsibility for safeguarding the health of the population. The act permitted localities to establish health boards, which could regulate practices and conditions deemed to harm health. The health boards could also manage sanitation, waste disposal, and burial grounds.

A contemporary of Edwin Chadwick's was John Snow (1813–1858), a medical doctor. Due to his work on cholera in 1854, he is widely considered to be the father of epidemiology. Snow was sceptical about the dominant miasma theory of disease transmission. By marking reported cases of cholera on a map, Snow discovered that water supplies were associated with an outbreak in the Soho area of London. He identified the source of the problem as being drinking water obtained from the Broad Street pump. He ordered the removal of the handle from the pump and thereby prevented further proliferation of the disease.

> **KEY POINT**
>
> Sanitary reform produced marked improvement in the health of the working population via dramatic falls in deaths from filth diseases such as cholera, smallpox, and typhoid.

The late 1800s saw dramatic advancements in bacteriology. The work of Louis Pasteur in the 1860s and Robert Koch in the 1880s and 1890s validated the germ theory of disease: that many diseases are caused by microorganisms. Germ theory became the dominant theory of disease, which in turn stimulated the development of antibiotics and highlighted the importance of hygienic practices. The discovery of penicillin in 1928 by Alexander Fleming heralded a new age of curative medicine (although usable quantities of the drug were not available until the 1940s).

The huge advances made by the public health movement from the 1850s to the 1950s began to see the burden of disease shift from acute, infectious illness that often killed in infancy to chronic diseases that manifested in middle age (such as heart disease and cancers).

> **KEY POINT**
>
> As the number of people succumbing to infectious disease at a young age fell, many more people began to suffer from chronic diseases that began in middle age.

By 1940 it had become apparent that the advances in health status described previously were not being enjoyed by all. There was little or no state support for those unable to work, and many poor people were unable to access medical help. Economist William Beveridge was asked to look into the haphazard social security system. The Beveridge Report, published in 1942, served as the basis for the reformist post-war Labour administration's welfare state, including the National Health Service (NHS).

 See Chapter 2 for more detail on the NHS.

The creation of the NHS in 1948 was seen as a major advance for public health in the UK. The new service was comprehensive, inclusive, and free at the point of delivery. For the first time, workers' dependents, the poor, and those requiring specialist services were able to access suitable health care. However, concerns were raised from the outset that the NHS was a sickness rather than a health service—that it was too focused on treatment rather than the prevention of ill health.

SELF CHECK 4.4

Why was the creation of the NHS viewed as a major advance for public health?

The 'new' public health

The term 'new public health' implies the rediscovery of and some continuity with the 'old' public health project (referring to nineteenth century public health). In 1974 Marc Lalonde, the then Canadian Minister for Health and Welfare, published a report entitled *A New Perspective on the Health of Canadians* (to become known as the *Lalonde Report*). It has been described (Hancock, 1986) as 'the first government document in the Western World to acknowledge that the current emphasis upon a biomedical health care system is not entirely desirable for the enhancement of health, nor particularly relevant to prevention.'

Lalonde suggested that future improvements in the health of Canadians would come mainly from improvements in the environment, moderating risky lifestyles, and increasing our understanding of human biology. Its intellectual inspiration came from the work of Thomas McKeown.

McKeown's critique of modern medicine and health care, *The Role of Medicine*, was first published in 1976. McKeown's argument was that medicine was too disease-focused and had a preoccupation with the individual at the expense of taking a more holistic view. He believed the emphasis placed on curative medicine as the prime driver in the reduction of mortality witnessed since the eighteenth century was misplaced. Economic growth, better standards of living, and improved nutrition were all more important than the role of medicine. McKeown's thesis served to focus attention on the wider causes of ill health and created a broader awareness of the social and environmental factors which affect health.

Health inequalities and the Black Report

The population of the UK has been classified according to occupation since 1851. In 1913 occupations were stratified into 'social classes'. These became known as the Registrar General's Social Classes (RGSC; renamed Social Class based on Occupation in 1990). Another classification system that is widely used by government departments and market researchers is the National Readership Survey (NRS) social grades. In the RGSC and NRS social grades, households were classified according to the occupation of the head of the household (the oldest male inhabitant). Since 2001, the primary social classification used by government departments in the UK has been the National Statistics Socioeconomic Classification (NS-SEC). In contrast to the older classifications, the NS-SEC uses the Household Reference Point (HRP). The HRP is the person responsible for owning or renting the property. In the case of joint householders, the person with the highest income becomes the HRP. Where incomes are equal, the oldest person is taken as the HRP. These classifications of social class are shown in Table 4.2.

Improvements in sanitation, road safety, medical knowledge, and technology, among other things, coupled with a reduction in poverty, meant that standards of health improved dramatically throughout the twentieth century. Standards of health are most commonly measured in terms of mortality rates and life expectancy. In the UK in 2009, life expectancy at birth for

TABLE 4.2 Commonly used classifications of social class in the UK

RGCS[1]		NRS[2] social grades		NS-SEC[3]	
Class	Occupational group	Class	Occupational group	Class	Occupational group
I	Professional occupations	A	Higher managerial, administrative or professional	1	Higher managerial, administrative, and professional occupations
II	Managerial and technical occupations	B	Intermediate managerial, administrative or professional	2	Lower managerial, administrative, and professional occupations
IIIN	Skilled non-manual occupations	C1	Supervisory or clerical and junior managerial, administrative or professional	3	Intermediate occupations
IIIM	Skilled manual occupations	C2	Skilled manual workers	4	Small employers and own-account workers
IV	Partly skilled occupations	D	Semi- and unskilled manual workers	5	Lower supervisory and technical occupations
V	Unskilled occupations	E	Casual or lowest grade workers, pensioners and others who depend on the welfare state for their income	6	Semi-routine occupations
				7	Routine occupations
				8	Never worked and long-term unemployed

[1]Registrar General's Social Classes (renamed Social Class based on Occupation in 1990).
[2]National Readership Survey.
[3]National Statistics Socioeconomic Classification.

women was 82 years, compared with 49 years in 1901; for men it was 78 years, compared with 45 years.

While the standard of health of all the population has improved over that time, the difference in health between the richest and the poorest members of society has widened dramatically; the poorest individuals in society suffer more ill health and die younger than their richer contemporaries. This is not to say that health differences are confined to differences between the poor and the rest of society. They run right through society, with every section of the social hierarchy having worse health than the level above it.

KEY POINT

The difference in health status between rich and poor is pronounced and has been widening consistently since the early 1970s.

In the mid to late 1970s a key area identified for future intervention by the government was inequalities in health status. A research working group on inequalities in health chaired by Sir Douglas Black (at that time the President of the Royal College of Physicians) was appointed. The subsequent report of this group (better known as the *Black Report*) was published in 1980.

The conclusion reached by the working group was that the poorer health experience of lower occupational groups applied at all stages of life, and that the class gradient in the UK seemed to be greater than in some comparable countries and was becoming more marked. Their research established that much of the problem lay outside the scope of the NHS. Numerous factors were involved, the majority of which were social and economic in nature. Income, employment status, the nature of employment, environment, education, housing, transport, and lifestyles all affect health and all favour the better off, in a number of different respects. In addition, despite being the group most likely to need the services of the health care system, the manual classes made less use of the NHS than the better off.

The *Black Report* made a total of 37 recommendations, including redressing the balance of the health care system to give more emphasis to prevention, primary care, and community health, and radically improving the material conditions of life for poorer groups, especially children and people with disabilities, by increasing or introducing certain cash benefits.

4.5 'Contemporary' public health policy and practice

Governments exert an influence on the health status of the populations that they govern via the policy process. Policies in whatever field—be that taxation, education, employment, social security, or pensions—can impact on health status. An example is provided in Figure 4.3, which shows that countries that restrain inequalities in wealth between the highest and lowest earners in society have healthier populations with fewer social problems (alcohol abuse, drug misuse, antisocial behaviour, etc.). Health policies—**White Papers**, legislative amendments, or entirely new pieces of legislation—influence the practice of health care professionals and how health care is provided, which can have a profound impact on the overall health of the population.

The political ideologies of ruling parties influence the policies they produce. A clear example of this was provided in the period immediately after the end of the Second World War. The post-war Labour administration of Prime Minister Clement Attlee was elected on a platform of social reform—the maintenance of full employment and the introduction of a 'cradle to grave' welfare state. Attlee appointed Aneurin Bevan, a committed **socialist**, as his Minster of Health. The National Health Service Act of 1946 was based largely on the socialist doctrine of: 'from each according to his ability to pay, to each according to his needs as a patient'. Bevan, writing in 1952, confirmed this stating: 'A free health service is pure socialism and as such it is opposed to the hedonism of capitalist society.'

Health strategies in the UK

The UK's first-ever health strategy, *Health of the Nation*, was published in 1992 with the stated aim of

FIGURE 4.3   Health and social problems are worse in more unequal countries (after Wilkinson and Pickett, 2009; reproduced with permission).

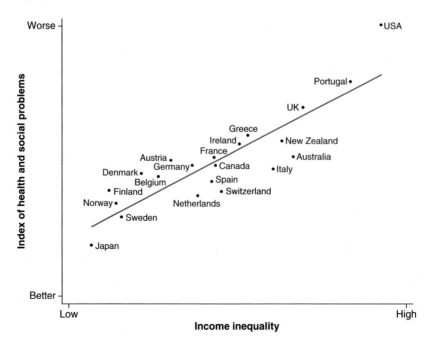

'[securing] continuing improvement in the general health of the population of England by: adding years to life ... and adding life to years'. This differed from previous health initiatives in that it adopted a strategic approach and, for the first time, focused managerial attention on the achievement of real health outcomes as opposed to improvements in health care processes such as waiting lists. In June 1999 *Health of the Nation* was replaced by a new strategy called *Saving Lives: Our Healthier Nation*. A key aim of the new strategy was the reduction of health inequalities. It is worth noting that, with the process of **devolution** well underway in the UK, this strategy was specific to England.

 See Chapter 2 for more information on how health care in the UK is organized.

The Public Health White Paper *Choosing Health: Making Healthy Choices Easier* was published in November 2004. It built on two government-commissioned reviews by Derek Wanless, which had highlighted the cost-effectiveness of focusing on public health. *Choosing Health* established what it described as three core principles of a new public health approach:

1. *Informed choice*: helping individuals to make informed decisions about choices that impact on their health.

2. *Personalization*: support to be tailored to the needs of the individual.

3. *Working together*: emphasizing the importance of partnerships across communities, including local government, the NHS, business, advertisers, retailers, the voluntary sector, faith groups, and many others.

Choosing Health also detailed six overarching priorities for action:

1. Reducing the number of people who smoke.

2. Reducing obesity and improving diet and nutrition.

3. Increasing exercise.

4. Encouraging and supporting sensible drinking.

5. Improving sexual health.

6. Improving mental health.

The priority areas and targets of all three of the strategies described in this section (*Health of the Nation; Saving Lives: Our Healthier Nation*; and *Choosing Health*) are shown in Table 4.3.

The UK General Election of 2010 resulted in a coalition government of Conservatives and Liberal Democrats. The coalition's proposals for NHS reform were outlined in the White Paper *Equity and Excellence: Liberating the NHS*. The proposed reforms were based on three principles:

1. Patients would be placed at the heart of the NHS. They would have more choice and control and more access to information on the performance of NHS services and professionals. Shared decision-making would become the norm, with 'no decision about me without me'.

2. There would be an increased focus on clinical outcomes such as cancer and stroke survival rates.

3. Health professionals would be empowered. Front-line staff would be given more control, with health care being run from the bottom up (that is, with decisions being made by professionals and their patients).

Liberating the NHS reiterated the government's commitment to the founding principles of the NHS—a comprehensive service, available to all, free at the point of use, and based on clinical need not the ability to pay—with the goal of creating an NHS which achieves results that are among the best in the world. The public health budget would be protected. It would be allocated according to population health outcomes, with an added premium to promote action to reduce health inequalities.

In an extension of New Labour's devolvement of NHS budgets to local NHS bodies (in England, primary care trusts (PCTs), which are responsible for the provision of primary care services within a specific area), the White Paper stated a desire to devolve commissioning to GPs, effectively abolishing PCTs. Local authorities would promote the integration of local NHS services, social care, and health improvement. All NHS trusts (bodies providing secondary care within the NHS; that is, hospitals) would become

TABLE 4.3 A summary of the key areas and targets for English health strategies

Priority areas	Health of the Nation[1]	Saving Lives: Our Healthier Nation[2]	Choosing Health: Making Healthy Choices Easier[3]
Coronary heart disease, stroke, and related illnesses	• Reduce the death rate in people aged under 65 years by 40% by 2000 • Reduce the death rate in people aged 65 to 74 years by 30% by 2000	• Reduce the death rate in people aged under 75 years by at least two-fifths	• Reduce the number of people who smoke • Reduce obesity and improve diet and nutrition • Increase exercise levels • Encourage and support sensible drinking
Accidents	• Reduce the death rate for accidents in those aged under 15 years by 33% by 2005 • Reduce the death rate for accidents in those aged 15 to 24 years by 25% by 2005 • Reduce the death rate for accidents in those aged 65 years and over by 33% by 2005	• Reduce the death rate from accidents by at least one-fifth and reduce the rate of serious injury by at least one-tenth	–
Cancer	• Reduce the death rate for breast cancer in women invited for screening by at least 25% by 2000 • Reduce the incidence of invasive cervical cancer by 20% by 2000 • Reduce the death rate for lung cancer in those aged under 75 years by 30% for men and 15% for women by 2010 • Halt the year-on-year increase in the incidence of skin cancer by 2005	• Reduce the death rate in people aged under 75 years by at least one-fifth	• Reduce the number of people who smoke • Reduce obesity and improve diet and nutrition • Increase exercise levels • Encourage and support sensible drinking
Mental illness	• Improve appreciably the health and social functioning of mentally ill people • Reduce the overall suicide rate by 15% by 2000 • Reduce the suicide rate of severely mentally ill people by 33% by 2000	• Reduce the death rate from suicide and undetermined injury by at least one-fifth	• Improve mental health
HIV/AIDS and sexual health	• Reduce the incidence of gonorrhoea by 20% by 1996 (as an indicator of HIV/AIDS trends) • Reduce the rate of conception in girls aged under 16 years by 50% by 2000	–	• Improve sexual health

[1]Department of Health, 1992. Strategy applicable to Scotland and Wales in addition to England.
[2]Department of Health, 1999.
[3]Department of Health, 2004.

foundation trusts (trusts with a greater degree of independence from Department of Health/NHS control). This would essentially place hospitals outside the direct control of the Department of Health. The power of ministers to influence the running of the NHS was to be limited. Monitor—the regulator of Foundation Trusts—would become an economic regulator, with a duty to promote competition between providers of health and social care. These changes constituted arguably the most extensive reorganiza-

tion of the structure of the NHS since its establishment in 1948.

Many of these proposals required primary legislation (in the form of a new Health and Social Care Bill) and parliamentary approval. The proposals were controversial, particularly around competition and the potential for increased private sector involvement in the provision of NHS services. The British Medical Association and the Royal College of Nursing (among other bodies) opposed the changes outlined in the first draft of the Health and Social Care Bill. Amidst strong opposition and following a 'listening exercise', numerous changes were made to the bill. The bill finally received Royal Assent in March 2012, becoming the Health and Social Care Act 2012.

The coalition's approach to public health was detailed in the White Paper *Healthy Lives, Healthy People*, which committed the government to 'protecting the population from serious health threats; helping people live longer, healthier and more fulfilling lives; and improving the health of the poorest, fastest'.

The White Paper maintained the explicit focus on empowering individuals, informed choice, and avoiding state intervention seen in *Choosing Health*. The document utilized Acheson's definition of public health yet stressed the necessity of working with the private sector to improve health outcomes. A key focus of the White Paper was 'nudge' theory: the idea that individuals can be nudged (for example, by increasing the prominence of healthy food in eateries) to adopt a healthier lifestyle rather than government having to intervene to influence behavioural change (by, for example, banning unhealthy practices). This policy was adopted despite the availability of very little evidence of the effectiveness of 'nudge' in improving health outcomes.

SELF CHECK 4.5

What is 'nudge' theory?

Healthy Lives, Healthy People also announced a 'public health responsibility deal' to work collaboratively with business and the voluntary sector in five areas: food, alcohol, physical activity, health at work, and behavioural change. This controversially gave companies such as fast-food retailers, processed drink manufacturers, and producers of alcoholic drinks a role in influencing government policy.

Devolution

Devolution, particularly the devolution of health care budgets, has led to the differential development of the NHS within each of the home countries. Each administration has developed country-specific health strategies. Table 4.4 lists these documents and notes any key advances for pharmacy within them. The strategic documents from the devolved administrations closely mirror developments within England. However, the market-based reforms pursued in England since 2000 have been largely rejected in Wales and Scotland. Another notable area of difference is the prominence afforded pharmacy in the health strategies of the devolved administrations.

TABLE 4.4 Post-devolution health strategies in the devolved administrations of the UK

Devolved administration	NHS policy document	Synopsis	Key developments for pharmacy
Scotland	*Partnership for Care*[1]	Pledged large increases in funding for the NHS. Services to become more patient-centred. Stressed the need for partnership working between patients, staff, and government.	Pledged to promote the use of local pharmacies as walk-in centres where people can receive health advice and services.
Wales	*Improving Health in Wales*[2]	NHS budget to be increased substantially. Highlighted the necessity for effective working across society to improve health status. Health inequalities identified as a key area for intervention.	Announced freezing of prescription charges and abolition of the prescription charge for those aged under 25 years.
Northern Ireland	*Investing for Health*[3]	Emphasis on partnership working among departments, public bodies, local communities, voluntary bodies, district councils, and the social partners to improve health status. Identified priority groups (the very young, the young, and the elderly) and priority topics (including smoking, physical activity, and sexual health).	Encouraged the development of 'health-promoting pharmacies'. Pharmacists working in these pharmacies would have the possibility to become involved in community outreach work. Premises would be able to be used for the provision of services by other health professionals.

[1]NHS Scotland, 2003.
[2]NHS Wales, 2001.
[3]Department of Health, Social Services and Public Safety, 2002.

4.6 The development of pharmacy's public health function

The practice of pharmacy in the UK changed markedly throughout the twentieth century, with the pharmacist's role changing from being client-facing to dispensary-focused and back to client-facing as the century progressed. Prior to 1948 pharmacists were to be found at the front of their shops with the responsibility for dispensing being left to the apprentices 'in the back'. The pharmacist was an important and well-known member of the local community—a readily available source of wisdom and advice about a whole range of health-related issues such as domestic hygiene, diet, and sexual health.

However, the provision of health-related advice was relegated in importance, practically overnight, with the arrival of the NHS in 1948. The volume of state prescriptions increased markedly. To meet this increased workload pharmacists relocated from 'front of house' to dispensary. The community pharmacist, at least in many places, virtually disappeared from the public's view, and hence its consciousness.

> SELF CHECK 4.6
>
> Why did the community pharmacist disappear from public view in the period after 1948?

Between the late 1940s and the 1970s the functions of the community pharmacist altered significantly in other ways. The responsibility for the making of medicines, a traditional role of pharmacists and their antecedents since the fifteenth century, was transferred to specialist manufacturers. Pharmacists no longer made something at the request of the patient, and instead simply supplied premanufactured products off the shelf.

 See Chapter 1 for more coverage of pharmacy's historical development.

By the late 1970s the profession itself realized that community pharmacy was in trouble:

One knew that there was a future for hospital pharmacists, one knew there was a future for industrial pharmacists, but one was not sure that one knew the future for the general practice pharmacist.

Source: *Pharmaceutical Journal*, 1981

Community pharmacists found themselves overtrained for what they did and under-utilized in relation to what they knew. The loss of pharmacy's traditional functions undermined its claim to professional status.

 See Chapter 2 for more discussion of the professional status of pharmacy.

The extended role and the public health function

The profession's response to the loss of its traditional functions was **role extension** as part of a movement toward 'reprofessionalization'. The traditional functions that pharmacy lost to industry (that is, drug procurement, storage, and compounding) fitted neatly into the 'technical paradigm'. With so few functions remaining in the technical paradigm, the process of reprofessionalization saw pharmacy gradually shift away from the technical paradigm toward an entirely different paradigm: one that emphasizes a disease- and patient-orientated approach to pharmaceutical decisions.

A significant part of the reprofessionalization of pharmacy took the form of a reclaiming of the pharmacist's traditional role in health promotion. In the early 1980s the first pharmacy-based health promotion schemes were launched. Topics covered included smoking cessation, healthy eating, alcohol awareness, and the safety of medicines. These were largely small-scale campaigns undertaken by a few committed pharmacists on a voluntary basis.

In 1986 the Nuffield Foundation published *Pharmacy: The Report of a Committee of Inquiry Appointed by the Nuffield Foundation* (the Nuffield Report), which supported the extended role of community pharmacists. Also in 1986 the 'Healthcare in the High Street' scheme was launched, involving the first national distribution of health education leaflets through pharmacy. The first government funding for the scheme was provided in 1989. Healthcare in the High Street was renamed 'Pharmacy Healthcare' and continued as a registered charity called PharmacyHealthLink before closing in 2011 after the government decided to withdraw its funding.

The Nuffield Report identified the fundamental problem of remuneration of the community pharmacist and its influence on their work, recognizing 'a clash between the promotion of what is professional and the requirements of running a business'. The report recommended that the basis of remuneration of community pharmacists should be changed. In particular it suggested that payments under the NHS pharmaceutical services contract in respect of prescriptions dispensed should be reduced, and separate payments made for other professional activities such as advice to patients and health education.

Pharmacy-specific government policy

The government policy paper *Pharmacy in the Future* was published in 2000. Reflecting the recommendations of the Nuffield Report, *Pharmacy in the Future* stated that the national contract for community pharmacies would be developed to reward high-quality services at the expense of those prepared only to provide the basic minimum. Furthermore, *Pharmacy in the Future* stated that pharmacists would spend more time focusing on the clinical needs of individual patients.

In England, pharmacy's potential public health role was finally recognized by government in 2003, with the publication of *A Vision for Pharmacy in the New NHS*.

The document described pharmacists as 'probably the biggest untapped resource for health improvement'. Included in the document were ten key roles for pharmacy, as identified by the then Chief Pharmaceutical Officer for England. One of the key roles was 'to be a public health resource and provide health promotion, health improvement and harm-reduction services'.

In an effort to tackle the underuse of pharmacy as a public health resource, the 2004 public health White Paper *Choosing Health* pledged to 'put in place measures which make the most of the contribution that pharmacists can make' and to publish a pharmaceutical public health strategy in 2005. *Choosing Health Through Pharmacy: A Programme for Pharmaceutical Public Health 2005–2015* was published in April 2005. The guidance identified public health targets on which pharmacists can have an impact, such as smoking, obesity, and sexual health, describes how pharmacists can become health champions by 2015, and provides examples of innovative service provision.

Pharmacy policy in the devolved administrations

While pharmacy's public health function did not receive significant attention in English policy until the mid 2000s, the roles that pharmacy could fulfil in public health were outlined robustly in pharmacy strategies in each of the devolved administrations in the early years of the new millennium and are detailed in Table 4.5. The specialism of pharmaceutical public health was embraced readily in Scotland and Wales, and pharmacy's position as a community resource was the subject of a policy document in Northern Ireland. This contrasted sharply with England, where the public health function of pharmacy was disjointed, with no coordinated pharmaceutical public health activity, a situation that has been somewhat rectified since 2005.

4.7 **Pharmacy's current public health function**

Pharmacists are involved in the maintenance of health and the prevention of ill health. They contribute daily to improving public health. This interaction occurs on two levels. Pharmacists on the 'front line' are involved in public health at a general level. At a more strategic level operate the 'specialists'. This section provides a

TABLE 4.5 Pharmacy strategies in the devolved administrations

Country	Pharmacy strategies and public health developments
Scotland	*The Right Medicine: A Strategy for Pharmaceutical Care in Scotland*[1] • Pharmacy's contribution to public health noted. • Pharmaceutical public health specifically identified as part of specialist public health practice. *Pharmacy for Health: The Way Forward for Pharmaceutical Public Health in Scotland*[2] • Specific pharmaceutical public health strategy. • Recognized pharmacists as public health practitioners but identified that their public health role had not yet been fully developed. • Pharmaceutical public health is not the exclusive domain of a small number of 'specialists' working in an NHS Board or academic department. Public health roles should extend across the breadth of the profession.
Wales	*Remedies for Success: A Strategy for Pharmacy in Wales*[3] • The emerging role of specialists in pharmaceutical public health (SiPPH) noted. • Stated that SiPPH have 'the potential to significantly improve the health of the population'. • SiPPH were to form part of a newly formed National Public Health Service.
Northern Ireland	*Making it Better: A Strategy for Pharmacy in the Community*[4] • Acknowledged that pharmacy is a key part of the community and that pharmacies can act as a vehicle for community empowerment, rather than just being an outlet. • Outlined plans for a 'Health-Promoting Pharmacies Network'. These pharmacies would be accredited and able to deliver public health services and messages as required by the local Health and Social Service Boards.

[1] Scottish Executive, 2001.
[2] Public Health Institute for Scotland, 2002.
[3] NHS Wales, 2002.
[4] Department of Health, Social Services and Public Safety, 2003.

brief overview of pharmacy's current involvement in public health.

The public health function of community pharmacists

Community pharmacists make a contribution to public health by providing appropriate information, advice, and support to the public on subjects ranging from contraception to medicines and alternative treatments to lifestyle. They also perform a useful 'signposting' role—referring patients to other appropriate health professionals and community organizations. In addition to this advisory function, a number of health-improving services are provided through pharmacies.

There is an evidence base on the effectiveness of community pharmacy-based public health interventions which demonstrates that community pharmacy can make a positive contribution to improving the public's health across a wide range of disease states, as well as reducing incidences of potentially health-damaging behaviours. Areas where pharmacy can contribute effectively include smoking cessation, hypertension, obesity, skin cancer prevention, drug misuse, diabetes, and sexual health. Examples of such interventions include:

- Smoking cessation services
- Weight management services (see Box 4.1)
- Needle exchange schemes
- Diabetes testing
- *Chlamydia* screening.

England and Wales

The contractual framework for NHS pharmaceutical services in England and Wales governs how community pharmacy contractors are remunerated for the provision of NHS services. (The Scottish contract has a different structure and is discussed elsewhere in this section). In 1994, health promotion became a contractual obligation for community pharmacy, with remuneration being received for the display of health promotion materials (posters and leaflets). This contractual obligation was consolidated in the 'new' contractual framework in 2005. The current

---

An example of a weight management service provided through community pharmacy (Coventry Weight Management Project)

A pilot weight management project commissioned by Coventry Teaching PCT has demonstrated that a pharmacy-based service can be effective in reducing participants' body mass index (BMI), a proxy measure of human body fat.

People were eligible to take part if they were over the age of 18 years with a BMI of at least 30 kg/m² and no more than 38 kg/m², with at least one additional risk factor : hypertension, type 2 diabetes, hyperlipidaemia, or an increased waist circumference (more than 102 cm for men, more than 88 cm for women).

At an initial consultation the pharmacist recorded height, weight, waist circumference, and, where appropriate, measured blood pressure and blood glucose. Participants were also provided with weight-loss advice materials and realistic targets were set for weight loss by the end of the programme. At follow-up appointments measurements were taken and more advice and support was provided.

Sixty-nine people completed Follow-up 4 (used for an interim analysis), with an average BMI reduction of 0.618 and an average reduction in waist circumference of 3.37 cm. Over two-thirds of participants in the project had lost weight.

---

contract consists of three different levels of service (see Table 4.6).

Public health was included in the essential services component of the contract. This is focused on the promotion of healthy lifestyles consisting of the provision of opportunistic advice to patients obtaining prescriptions from the pharmacy and involvement in public health campaigns. Many other harm-reducing and health-improving measures were included in the enhanced services section, including substance misuse, the provision of emergency hormonal contraception, smoking cessation, and needle exchange services.

KEY POINT

Public health is a contractual obligation for community pharmacists. Health promotion and lifestyle advice are essential services, with many other public health services located in the enhanced services section of the contract.

SELF CHECK 4.7

What are the three different levels of the community pharmacy contract for England and Wales and in which level does public health appear?

Scotland

The pharmaceutical services contract for Scotland has a different structure to its English equivalent. It has four distinct core components rather than differing levels of service:

- *Acute Medication Service*: the dispensing of prescriptions for acute conditions.

- *Chronic Medication Service*: the pharmaceutical contribution to the management of long-term conditions, allowing continuity of pharmaceutical care between the patient and their general practitioner, their practice team, and their community pharmacist.

- *Public Health Service*: the contribution of community pharmacists to improving health.

- *Minor Ailments Service*: the management of minor ailments through the NHS by community pharmacists.

In addition to the four core components there are also a number of additional services, such as out-of-hours services and harm-reduction services, with national benchmark specifications and remuneration rates which can be commissioned by local NHS Boards (similar to the enhanced service level of the contract in England).

TABLE 4.6 **The structure of the pharmacy contract**

Essential[1]	Advanced[2]	Enhanced and local[3]
Dispensing of medicines	Medicines Use Review and Prescription Intervention Service	Supervised administration of medicines
Repeat dispensing	Appliance Use Review Service	Needle and syringe exchange
Supply of appliances	Stoma Appliance Customization Service	On-demand availability of specialist drugs (for example, palliative care)
Waste management	New Medicine Service[4]	Stop smoking
Public health		Care-home service
Signposting		Medicines assessment and compliance support
Support for self-care		Medication review (full clinical review)
Clinical governance		Minor Ailment Service
		Out-of-hours service
		Supplementary prescribing
		Emergency hormonal contraception
		Seasonal influenza vaccination
		Patient group directions
		Chlamydia screening and treatment
		NHS Health Check (vascular risk assessment)
		Weight management
		Alcohol screening and brief intervention
		Anticoagulant management
		Independent prescribing
		Sharps disposal
		Emergency supply at NHS expense

[1]Offered by all contractors.
[2]Optional and require accreditation.
[3]The specification and value of these services are agreed nationally; however, they are commissioned locally by primary care trusts on the basis of need. Primary care trusts are also free to develop their own local services in response to identified need. This list is therefore indicative and is based on the template service specifications (including draft specifications) available on the Pharmaceutical Services Negotiating Committee's website: <http://www.psnc.org.uk/pages/enhanced_and_local_services.html>.
[4]This service was implemented from 1 October 2011.

Pharmacy in England

The 2008 pharmacy White Paper *Pharmacy in England* outlined how the current strengths of pharmacy could be built on in the future to deliver safe and effective patient-centred pharmaceutical services. In a continuation of the agenda of the previous 10 years, the strategy aimed to further the role extension of community pharmacists by supporting a shift in focus from dispensing to clinical services. Echoing Wanless, *Pharmacy in England* stated a desire to see pharmacists and pharmacies engaged in the drive to combat health inequalities and focusing on prevention as much as sickness.

 See 'Health strategies in the UK', in Section 4.5, for more about the Wanless reports.

The document contained some notable developments relevant to the public health function of community pharmacists, including the involvement of community pharmacy in the provision of vascular checks (see Box 4.2 for an example). This was to be a single, universal, integrated check, measuring the risk of cardiovascular disease, diabetes, and chronic kidney disease for all people aged 40–74 years. Vascular disease accounts for the largest part of health inequalities in England, with the burden falling disproportionately on the socioeconomically deprived and on certain ethnic groups (for example, South Asians). It was estimated that the scheme, to be provided in a variety of settings, would each year prevent:

- 9500 heart attacks and strokes
- 2000 deaths
- 4000 people developing diabetes.

Pharmacy in England also detailed how community pharmacies were to be repositioned, recognized, and valued as 'healthy living' centres (see Box 4.3). This would strengthen pharmacy's contribution to public health by making the pharmacy an expert health resource close to the patient's home and would exploit pharmacies' ready availability in deprived areas to expand access to health care. Pharmacists would focus on:

- promoting healthy living, health literacy, and supporting self-care;

BOX 4.2

An example of a vascular check provided through community pharmacies ('Heart MOT' service in South Birmingham PCT)

A service provided through 23 community pharmacies in Birmingham has demonstrated that pharmacies can successfully provide a cardiovascular risk assessment service that can attract men and provide access for classically hard-to-reach groups (individuals from deprived communities and Black and Asian communities).

Individuals aged between 40 and 70 years without known cardiovascular disease (CVD) were eligible for the service. Promotional materials encouraged individuals to visit a pharmacy for a 'Heart MOT', which measured and communicated the risk of developing CVD over the next 10 years. This took into account multiple risk factors including gender, age, ethnicity, cholesterol levels, blood glucose, blood pressure, and waist circumference. Family history of CVD and lifestyle history were also recorded.

Of 1130 clients, 60% were male, 25% were from the Asian community, and 7% were from the Black community. Overall, 70% of clients were referred to their general practice for follow-up: 18% of these with a CVD risk of at least 20% over the next 10 years, the remainder with individual risk factors.

BOX 4.3

An example of how community pharmacies can act as 'healthy living' centres (Portsmouth Healthy Living Pharmacies initiative)

NHS Portsmouth implemented a 'Healthy Living Pharmacy' (HLP) framework across the city. The aim of the project was to reduce health inequalities and prevent disease through the promotion of healthy lifestyles. NHS Portsmouth also wanted to increase public confidence in pharmacy by raising awareness of the expertise of pharmacists and their staff.

HLPs offered proactive well-being advice, accessible support for self-care, and support for people on medicines for long-term conditions. They also encouraged the use of various services in target groups such as smoking cessation, weight management, emergency hormonal contraception, and targeted medicines use reviews for those with asthma. HLPs also provided a minor ailments service.

HLPs were well received by the people of Portsmouth and demonstrated their effectiveness in improving respiratory function and decreasing the numbers of smokers. They made a real difference by consistently delivering high-quality services and advice. The HLP concept has since been rolled out to other areas of the country and research is being undertaken to assess its effectiveness in delivering positive health outcomes.

- providing opportunistic and prescription-linked healthy lifestyle advice;
- other public health initiatives such as involvement in immunization programmes;
- prevention as much as treatment.

The public health function of hospital pharmacists

Hospital pharmacists undertake numerous activities that contribute to the prevention of ill health. Changes to drug therapy are common in the hospital setting and a patient's medicines are routinely reconciled on transfer within the hospital setting and upon discharge. This medicines reconciliation activity reduces the possibility of errors occurring in the course of an individual's drug therapy. Hospital pharmacists also have an important role in promoting adherence to newly prescribed medication regimes.

A traditional function of hospital pharmacy has been the provision of drug information to health professional colleagues across all health care sectors. Such information promotes the safe and effective use of medications and helps to reduce the possibility of harm from adverse drug reactions. Hospital pharmacists also undertake strategic roles within secondary care, including involvement in audits of drug usage and membership of drugs and therapeutics committees promoting the evidence-based use of medicines.

Specialism in pharmaceutical public health

The public health function of pharmacists we have described can be defined as 'generalist' practice. However, in an agenda led mainly by the devolved administrations, pharmacists can attain specialist status, becoming specialists in pharmaceutical public health (SiPPHs).

Most front-line pharmacists working in health care settings already support the delivery of the public health agenda in some way. However, specialists work at a strategic or senior management level. They provide pharmacy-related input into strategic decision-making within public health departments, primarily within PCTs and their equivalents in the devolved administrations. Their unique contribution comes from specialist pharmaceutical expertise, experience of providing health services, and clinical practice.

SiPPHs are involved in both health protection and service planning. Their contribution is important in areas such as immunization programmes (particularly pandemic influenza planning), planning for the provision of pharmacy services in an emergency (such as a terrorist incident), and drug misuse. SiPPHs also have a role in coordinating the provision of services by their colleagues in the community.

 See Section 4.8 for more detail on pandemic influenza and terrorism.

4.8 Future health challenges and barriers to effective public health measures

Global health

The health challenges faced by developing nations are markedly different to those faced by developed nations. The World Bank categorizes nations into four bands based on income per person (gross national product (GNP) per capita): high income (for example, the UK: GNP per capita = $35 980), upper middle income (for example, Mexico: GNP per capita = $7835), lower middle income (for example, Thailand: GNP per capita = $3719) and low income (for example, Kenya: GNP per capita = $737). In 2008, 58% of deaths in low-income countries were due to communicable diseases (such as diarrhoeal diseases and infections), maternal and perinatal conditions, and nutritional deficiencies. This compares with just 7% of deaths from these causes in high-income countries. Conversely, the burden of death from non-communicable diseases (such as cancers and cardiovascular disease) is disproportionately elevated in high-income countries: 87% of all deaths in high-income countries are due to non-communicable disease compared with 33% of all deaths in low-income countries (see Figure 4.4).

In the developing world, life expectancy is directly linked to GNP per capita. This is a measure of absolute income. As GNP per capita increases, so does life expectancy. The relationship between GNP per capita and life expectancy ceases to exist once a certain level of GNP is reached. At this point, referred to by Wilkinson (1996) as 'the epidemiological transition', economies have advanced beyond a crucial stage when living standards reach a threshold level adequate to ensure basic material standards for all, and cancers and degenerative diseases overtake infectious diseases as the main cause of death.

> **KEY POINT**
>
> The epidemiological transition is the point within a country where the economy has advanced to such a point that chronic disease overtakes infectious disease as the main cause of death.

> **SELF CHECK 4.8**
>
> What are the major causes of death in low-income countries and how does this differ from high-income countries?

Health challenges in low-income countries

A key reason for this difference in disease burden between high- and low-income countries is the disparity in life expectancy between low-income (primarily located in sub-Saharan Africa) and high-income countries (primarily located in Western Europe and North America). Life expectancy at birth in low-income countries is 57 years, compared with 80 years in high-income countries.

> **KEY POINT**
>
> With life expectancies so low in low-income countries, individuals frequently do not live long enough to develop chronic, non-communicable diseases.

The world is in the grip of a global pandemic of human immunodeficiency virus/acquired immunodeficiency syndrome (HIV/AIDS). In 2008, in

75

FIGURE 4.4 Burden of disease by World Bank income group (2008). Data from WHO Global Health Observatory Data Repository at <http://apps.who.int/ghodata/>.

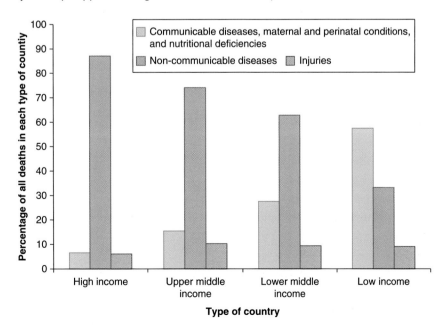

excess of 33 million people worldwide were living with HIV/AIDS. This burden was borne overwhelmingly by low-income countries in sub-Saharan Africa (22.4 million). In Botswana, for example, a quarter of the population aged 15–49 years had HIV, and 8% of all deaths in low-income countries were attributable to HIV/AIDS. Antiretroviral drugs have proved effective at slowing the progress of the infection and lengthening the lives of those living with HIV. While access to antiretroviral therapy in low- and middle-income countries has increased markedly—a 10-fold increase between 2003 and 2008—coverage in sub-Saharan Africa remains limited (only 44% of people in need of antiretroviral therapy were estimated to be receiving such services in 2008). Despite the significant gains accomplished during the previous decade, the HIV epidemic in sub-Saharan Africa continues to outpace the response.

A further 8% of deaths in low-income countries are caused by diarrhoeal diseases. Approximately 2.5 million people every year die from diarrhoeal diseases and nearly 1 in 5 child deaths (approximately 1.5 million each year) are due to diarrhoea. It has been estimated that 88% of that burden is attributable to unsafe water supply, poor sanitation, and lack of hygiene. Over 1 billion people globally have no access to safe drinking water, and 2.4 billion people do not have access to acceptable sanitation facilities. Diarrhoea is easily treatable but only 39% of children in developing countries receive the recommended treatment.

Another major killer in the developing world is malaria. The disease is caused by *Plasmodium spp.* parasites that are transmitted to people through the bites of infected mosquitoes. In 2009 there were 225 million cases of malaria and 781 000 deaths. Most of these deaths occurred among children in Africa, where the disease accounts for 20% of all childhood deaths. The disease is both preventable and treatable. It can be prevented by the use of mosquito nets impregnated with insecticide (or by drugs for travellers to endemic areas) and treated effectively by drugs. Since 2008 there has been a concerted drive by the WHO to increase the coverage of effective prevention measures. Between 2008 and 2010 almost 300 million mosquito nets were delivered to sub-Saharan Africa,

enough to protect nearly 600 million people. Access to effective treatment remains limited, however.

Effective public health interventions could prevent many of these deaths. However, coverage is uniformly low and health care systems are substandard and under-resourced. Money for health care is scarce. There is an estimated shortage of approximately 4.3 million doctors, midwives, nurses, and support workers worldwide, with that shortage being most severe in the poorest countries, particularly in sub-Saharan Africa, where the need for health workers is greatest.

> **KEY POINT**
>
> Many deaths in low-income countries could be prevented by relatively simple public health interventions such as the provision of clean drinking water.

Health challenges in the UK

The focus of public health interventions in the UK, and in almost all developed nations, is now placed on chronic diseases (the most prevalent of which are cardiovascular diseases, cancers, respiratory diseases, and diabetes) and health-damaging behaviours. These areas have been the focus of successive health strategies in the UK. As detailed in *Healthy Lives, Healthy People* the UK is now the most obese nation in Europe. Rates of sexually transmitted infections are high, as are rates of problem drug use and alcohol abuse. Despite the relatively high level of attention given to health inequalities over the last 30 years, health inequalities between rich and poor have been getting progressively worse.

> **KEY POINT**
>
> Most public health interventions in the UK are focused on reducing rates of chronic diseases such as CVD and cancers.

 See Section 4.5 for details of these strategies.

While there is a role for public health in combating all chronic diseases and health-damaging behaviours, obesity has been highlighted as one of the foremost health issues facing the UK today. Obesity is now a global problem but its prevalence is higher in developed nations. In England in 2007 24% of adults were obese. This has been forecast to rise to over 50% by 2050, with a corresponding cost to the NHS of £9.7 billion. Individual-level interventions are unlikely to be successful in combating this surge in obesity prevalence. A population-level approach focused on prevention is necessary, including the promotion of healthy diets, a cultural change in attitudes towards diet and activity, and modification of the built environment to encourage more walking, jogging, cycling etc.

Case Study 4.1 describes how a pharmacist could help an individual with obesity avoid long-term health problems.

Some emerging global threats

In 2009, a pandemic of influenza (the H1N1 version of the influenza virus) swept across the world. This was a new virus, emanating from animals, to which many people had no pre-existing immunity. The pandemic began in April and, by June, 30 000 cases had been reported in 74 countries. In October 2009 the UK began vaccinating its health care workers and vulnerable patient groups (such as pregnant women, young children, and those with pre-existing respiratory illness) against the virus. In August 2010 the WHO announced that the H1N1 influenza virus had moved into the post-pandemic period. The threat from this pandemic and potentially new pandemics of influenza (such as avian influenza H5N1) remain. It is therefore important that countries remain vigilant and alert for outbreaks and continue to take measures to protect their populations against influenza.

Climate change also constitutes an emerging threat to public health. A warmer climate may lead to increased levels of some air pollutants and a more variable climate threatens to increase the hazards of extreme weather. In addition, many of the major killers, including cholera and malaria, are climate sensitive as regards rainfall and temperature. In *Pharmacy in England*, pharmacists were identified as individuals who could take a lead in helping to combat climate change by promoting sustainable development. Community pharmacies are an integral part of local communities and community pharmacists are trusted professionals who are in an ideal position to take a lead on sustainable development by, for example, promoting active transport (cycling, running, walking). The promotion of active transport will improve physical health, reduce obesity levels, improve air quality (as there will be a reduction in emissions from motorized transport), and therefore reduce the incidence of respiratory illness.

Since 11 September 2001, renewed attention has been focused on terrorism as a threat to public health. Terrorist acts have the potential to cause sudden, unexpected, and dramatic increases in injuries and deaths. Of particular concern has been a perceived risk of the use of highly infectious agents such as anthrax and smallpox in an explosive device (a so-called 'dirty bomb'), with the potential to cause large-scale death and disease. Planning by government bodies has been intensified to protect health in such circumstances.

Barriers to effective public health measures

Historically, public health strategies have failed to resolve philosophical tensions that have endured for centuries; namely, what is the balance that should be struck between intervention by the state and individual freedom?

Such tensions were evident during the Victorian cholera outbreaks, when a leader in *The Times* stated: 'We prefer to take our chances with cholera and the rest than be bullied into good health.' Since the publication of the UK's first health strategy in 1992, governments have feared criticism of running a 'nanny state' and have largely avoided direct regulation wherever possible; the foreword to the latest public health strategy states: 'The dilemma for government is this: it is simply not possible to promote healthier lifestyles through Whitehall diktat and nannying about the way people should live.'

Alan is 57 years old and looking forward to retiring from his job as an insurance broker. He is aware that he has gained weight over a number of years and that his weight increased more rapidly after he tore the cartilage in his right knee whilst refereeing a rugby match (causing his retirement from the game) a couple of years ago. He had meant to join the local gym or take up tennis but had not quite got around to doing it. He was looking forward to all the time he would have to get fit again once he had retired, as the most daily exercise he did was walk to and from the station to catch the train to work—about 300 yards from his front door.

Alan realized that he was starting to get breathless when he walked upstairs and that he had developed varicose veins. He noticed that he frequently suffered from gastro-oesophageal reflux after eating and had started to complain to his wife Barbara that he often just did not feel well. Barbara, a slim woman in her mid 50s, encouraged him to go and have a check-up and he subsequently booked himself into the well-person clinic run by the pharmacist at his local pharmacy.

Catherine, the pharmacist, started the check-up by chatting to Alan about his general health. She asked whether there was any family history of heart disease or strokes and discovered that he was not currently taking any medicines. Alan replied that his father had died of a heart attack when he was aged 68 years and his mother had died following a stroke at 62 years.

The pharmacist asked Alan about his current eating and exercise habits and Alan explained about the knee injury and the knock-on effects from that. He admitted that he enjoyed a fried breakfast, enjoyed a canteen-cooked lunch of two courses and a cooked dinner plus dessert. The pharmacist asked if he snacked during the day and Alan said: 'No, but I do have a chocolate bar with my mid-morning coffee and I like to have a pint or two of lager later in the evening, often with a bag of crisps.'

Catherine weighed Alan (95 kg) and measured his height (1.75 m) and waist circumference (93 cm).

REFLECTION QUESTIONS

1. Individuals are classed as obese when their BMI is 30 kg/m^2 or more. Calculate Alan's BMI using the following formula:

$$BMI = \frac{Weight\ (kg)}{(Height\ (m))^2}$$

2. Alan's BMI indicates that he is obese. Guidance on obesity from the National Institute of Health and Clinical Excellence outlines that attempts should initially be made to modify Alan's lifestyle. What advice could you offer Alan?

3. It has been suggested that an increased proportion of pharmacists' time is likely to be spent on attempting to combat obesity in the future. Why might this be true?

Answers

1. $BMI = \frac{95}{(1.75)^2} = \frac{95}{3.06} = 31\ kg/m^2$

2.
- Obesity is caused by taking in more energy than is expended over a period of time.
- If Alan lost weight he would immediately start reducing the risks of the other conditions associated with obesity.
- Stress that obesity is a condition that Alan himself could have some control over by eating a balanced diet and increasing his exercise.
- Dietary advice:
  - Base meals on starchy foods.
  - Eat lots of fruit and vegetables.
  - Eat more fish (including a portion of oily fish per week).
  - Eat less saturated fat and sugar.
  - Eat less salt (maximum of 6 g daily in adults).
  - Drink plenty of water.
  - Don't skip breakfast.
  - Enjoy your food.
- Alan should also be advised to increase his level of physical activity. It is recommended that adults undertake at least 30 min of at least moderate-intensity physical activity on five or more days a week. Examples of moderate-intensity activity include brisk walking, cycling, swimming, and stair climbing.

3. Obesity has been highlighted as one of the foremost health challenges facing the nation today. Around a quarter of adults in England are obese and this proportion is forecast to grow to over 50% by 2050. An increased BMI makes it more likely that an individual will suffer from a wide range of chronic conditions, including osteoarthritis, cardiovascular disease, type 2 diabetes, and various cancers.

Instead, particularly since 2004, successive govern-ments have placed the onus on providing information and support to enable individuals to make healthy choices for themselves. Doubts have been raised that such a prominent focus on the individual can be effec-tive in tackling the challenges faced by government, particularly the challenges posed by health inequali-ties and obesity.

Ever since the development of the first health strate-gies in developed nations in the 1970s, pressure has been placed on governments to critically examine their health care systems. The emphasis placed on pro-moting efficiency within the NHS since the late 1970s has focused attention on how to best use the finite resources allocated for health care by central govern-ment. This, in turn, demands that the health care pro-vided by the NHS is cost-effective.

Strategies aimed at the prevention of ill health often lack evidence of cost-effectiveness. While such strate-gies may be expected to reduce the burden of treat-ment on the NHS, they may also have longer-term costs that impact on public services in the future. For example, if strategies to reduce alcohol consumption are successful we may expect to see a reduction in hos-pital admissions and mortality rates owing to alcohol intake. While this may lead to an overall reduction in health care costs it may also lead to an increase in the costs of pensions and long-term care.

The drive for efficiency allied to the rise of a tar-get-driven culture within the NHS goes some way to explaining why a perception exists that public health has been pushed to the margins of contemporary health policy. It is much easier to measure improve-ments in service delivery than achieve well-being in specific population groups, which may explain why much health policy has a downstream focus on symp-toms and treatments and changing people's behaviour and lifestyles, not conditions or places.

 See Section 4.5 for more information on public health policy and practice.

Barriers to pharmacy's involvement in the new public health agenda

The current public health practice of community pharmacists is focused on downstream interventions such as health promotion, not on public health in its widest sense. Pharmacists tend to focus on individual behaviour; that is, lifestyles, with little consideration of wider population-level determinants of both health and behaviour—an attitude possibly linked with phar-macy's strong adherence to a biomedical model of health and illness.

Community pharmacists have often been described as the most accessible of health professionals. This accessibility can, at least in part, be attributed to the operation of community pharmacies in a retail envi-ronment. While approximately 80% of a community pharmacy's turnover may be derived from the con-tracted provision of NHS services (the core dispensing function), pharmacies can only continue to function while they are profitable. This context has fostered a tension between the desire of pharmacists to provide a health service and the necessity to operate a profitable business and, to some eyes, attempting to 'graft' a pub-lic health mindset onto pharmacists operating within a commercial environment is contradictory.

Within pharmacy there is frequently a low level of cooperation between the fragmented and isolated sections that make up the profession, be it between hospital pharmacists and community pharmacists, community pharmacists and primary care pharmacists, or within the community pharmacy sector, where contractors are often divided by the need to seek a competitive advantage. Such divisions run contrary to a public health approach that is both collectivist and multidisciplinary in nature.

KEY POINT

Pharmacy contractors operate in a commercial environment and are divided by the need to seek competitive advantage. This may make it difficult for pharmacists to develop a public health mindset.

CHAPTER SUMMARY

➤ Health is a state of complete physical, mental, and social well-being and not merely the absence of disease or infirmity.

➤ Public health is focused on the health states of populations rather than individuals.

➤ Public health is the science and art of preventing disease, prolonging life, and promoting, protecting, and improving health through organized efforts of society.

➤ Sanitary reform in the late nineteenth and early twentieth centuries led to a marked improvement in the health of the population via dramatic falls in communicable diseases.

➤ In many parts of the world, communicable diseases are still the primary cause of death and disease.

➤ As economies develop, the burden of disease moves from infectious diseases to chronic disease such as cancers and cardiovascular disease.

➤ As the burden of disease moves from infectious to chronic disease, the focus of the public health movement changes to reflect this.

➤ The creation of the NHS meant that workers' dependents and the poor could access health care for the first time.

➤ A key focus of the new public health approach is on health inequalities. Such inequalities run right through society, with each section of the social hierarchy having worse health than the level above it.

➤ Since the Black Report in 1980, health inequalities have continued to widen.

➤ The UK has had a series of health strategies since 1992. While these have all differed they also share a number of similarities.

➤ Community pharmacy practice, and with it community pharmacy's public health function, changed markedly throughout the twentieth century.

➤ Pharmacy's public health function has been developed as part of a move towards role extension in response to the loss of its traditional function.

➤ The public health function of community pharmacists is focused on downstream individual-level service provision and health promotion.

➤ There are barriers to both improving public health and developing pharmacy's public health function.

FURTHER READING

Calman, K. The 1848 Public Health Act and its relevance to improving public health in England now. *British Medical Journal* 1998; 317: 596–8.

This article highlights the importance of the 1848 Act and how it is still relevant today.

Navarro, V. and Shi, L. The political context of social inequalities and health. *Social Science and Medicine* 2001; 52: 481–91.

This article demonstrates how political ideologies can influence the health status of populations.

Crowley, P. and Hunter, D.J. Putting the public back into public health. *Journal of Epidemiology and Community Health* 2005; 59: 265–7.

> This article provides a critical perspective on public health policy in the early New Labour period.

Anderson, S. Community pharmacy and public health in Great Britain, 1936 to 2006: How a phoenix rose from the ashes. *Journal of Epidemiology and Community Health* 2007; 61: 844–8.

> This article provides a historical overview of community pharmacy's contribution to public health.

Jesson, J. and Bissell, P. Public health and pharmacy: A critical review. *Critical Public Health* 2006; 16: 159–69.

> This article offers a sociological critique of community pharmacy's contribution to public health and highlights some of the barriers that prevent pharmacy from fulfilling its potential in public health.

Prescribing and dispensing

SUE C. JONES

So far in this text we have covered strategic areas of pharmacy, from the inception of the profession through to how pharmacy fits in with the wider scope of health care provision in the UK. As you have seen from Chapter 3, pharmacy is a highly regulated profession with many laws affecting its practice. Similarly, from its roots in professionalism, a code of conduct allows pharmacists to consider ethical matters using their professional expertise and judgement. The purpose of this chapter is to consider what happens when a patient sees a prescriber and is given a prescription to be dispensed in the pharmacy. Prescribing and dispensing take place in primary and secondary care, and while the processes involved are largely similar, there are some differences in terms of the prescription forms. This chapter will focus on prescribing and dispensing in primary care.

Learning objectives

Having read this chapter you are expected to be able to:

➤ Map a patient's journey from their prescriber to their medication being dispensed.

➤ Describe the restrictions placed on the different professions eligible to become prescribers.

➤ Explore the legal, clinical, ethical, and economic factors that need to be considered when writing a prescription for a patient.

➤ Describe the clinical checks that are required as part of the dispensing process.

➤ Describe the legal framework within which prescriptions are screened prior to dispensing.

➤ Explore the ethical perspectives that may be encountered when a prescription is dispensed.

➤ List the ways in which medicines can be extemporaneously prepared for the patient.

➤ Describe the checks that should be completed to confirm the accuracy of dispensed medicines against prescriptions (to reduce the risk of medication errors).

➤ Define adherence and explore how pharmacists can promote concordance.

➤ Understand the nature of the information that patients may require in order to make a decision about their medication-taking behaviour, including patient counselling and advice.

5.1 The journey of a patient from prescriber to medicine

There are a number of steps that must be completed before medicines can be given to patients with acute or chronic medical conditions who require treatment. Figure 5.1 illustrates the steps involved when a patient with an acute medical complaint presents for diagnosis and treatment. There is considerable overlap between prescribing and dispensing with regard to

ensuring that the medicine is appropriate and safe for the patient. This overlap of roles and responsibilities is not an unnecessary duplication but is an integral part of the quality control process, which includes double checking to ensure medicines are used appropriately and safely. In this chapter each of these steps will be explored in detail.

5.2 Who can prescribe?

At the inception of the National Health Service (NHS) in 1948, prescribing was limited to physicians. As time has progressed the range of other health care professionals (HCP) able to prescribe has grown, although there may be limitations on what they can prescribe. Dentists can prescribe, at NHS expense, a limited number of medicines from a list called the Dental Practitioners' Formulary (DPF) which can be found in the *British National Formulary* (*BNF*). In the late 1990s community nurses who had successfully completed the appropriate additional training were

allowed to prescribe a limited range of medicines and appliances from the *Nurse Prescribers' Formulary*, (*NPF*) which can also be found in the *BNF*. In 2003 a new type of prescribing was introduced that created two types of prescriber: the independent prescriber and the supplementary prescriber.

Supplementary prescribers

Supplementary prescribers are not responsible for diagnosis but take responsibility for the ongoing care of the

FIGURE 5.1   From symptom to treatment: the patient journey

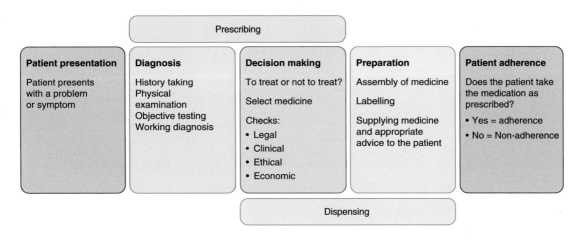

patient. Supplementary prescribing is a voluntary partnership between the independent prescriber (medical doctor) and the supplementary prescriber, who could be a pharmacist. Supplementary prescribers work within the remit of a document called a **clinical management plan (CMP)**. The CMP is specific to an individual patient and directs the conditions and medicines the supplementary prescriber can take responsibility for managing. There are some differences in terms of what can be prescribed between NHS and privately funded prescriptions and these are described in Table 5.1.

 See Chapter 2 for more on the NHS and private health care.

The range of professions from which supplementary prescribers can be drawn now includes all registered nurses, pharmacists, chiropodists, optometrists, physiotherapists, and radiographers. Members of these professions do not automatically become able to prescribe at registration. They must have the required amount of post-qualification experience and have successfully completed the appropriate prescribing training programme.

Independent prescribers

Nurses were the first non-medical profession able to qualify as independent prescribers. In 2006 pharmacists became eligible to train as non-medical prescribers and they were joined more recently by optometrists. It is likely that the number of professions able to become independent prescribers will continue to expand. Independent non-medical prescribers are not restricted in terms of what they can prescribe but they must be aware of their areas of professional competence and ensure that they work within the limitations of this competence. There are some differences in terms of what can be prescribed between NHS and privately funded prescriptions and these are described in Table 5.2.

What is a prescription?

It is important to consider the piece of paper that is produced to instruct the pharmacy about the patient's treatment. There are a range of prescription types available that may be issued by prescribers working in the community or hospital, and there are differences between the different parts of the UK. For an up-to-date list you should consult the website for the appropriate organization (see the 'Further reading' section). Generally, a prescription is a legal document that needs to contain all of the relevant information for the pharmacist to dispense the item and counsel the patient about its use. An example of a common NHS prescription is reproduced in Figure 5.2 and we will use this to illustrate the rest of the prescribing and dispensing process. Hospital inpatients rarely receive an actual prescription form but the information required is instead written on the patient's drug chart and this allows medicines to be supplied or administered to the patient.

Community pharmacists also manage minor ailments over the counter and this has been termed 'counter prescribing'. Obviously there is no written prescription when a community pharmacist is counter prescribing; but the points made in this chapter around clinical, ethical, and economic perspectives still apply. Legal perspectives also apply but the regulations differ.

TABLE 5.1 Summary of supplementary prescribing

Practitioner	Prescribed on NHS	Prescribed privately

Pharmacist, midwife, registered nurse, chiropodist/podiatrist, physiotherapist, radiographer, optometrist	• Any drug provided it is not blacklisted[1] and it is specified in the clinical management plan, including:
	  • Controlled drugs
	  • Unlicensed medicines
	• Any appliance that is in the Drug Tariff[1]
		• Any drug provided it is specified in the clinical management plan, including
		  • Controlled drugs
		  • Unlicensed medicines
		• Any appliance

[1]The blacklist and the Drug Tariff apply in primary care only. The 'blacklist' refers to a range of medicines, such as hypnotics and anxiolytics, that cannot be prescribed by brand name.

TABLE 5.2 Summary of independent prescribing

Practitioner	Prescribed on NHS	Prescribed privately
Doctor	• Any drug provided it is not blacklisted[2] • Any appliance that is in the Drug Tariff[2]	• Any drug • Any appliance
Dentist	• Only items specified in the Dental Practitioners' Formulary	• Any drug (professional body limits to dental treatment)
Community nurse[1]	• Drugs listed in the *Nurse Prescribers' Formulary* • Appliances in Drug Tariff[2]	• Drugs listed in the *Nurse Prescribers' Formulary* • Any appliance
Nurse prescriber[1]	• *Non-controlled drugs*: Any medicine provided it is not blacklisted[2] • *Controlled drugs*: Schedule 2, 3, 4, and 5—are not able to prescribe diamorphine, dipipanone, or cocaine for treating addiction but may prescribe these items for treating organic disease or injury	• *Non-controlled drugs: Any medicine* • *Controlled drugs*: Schedule 2, 3, 4, and 5—are not able to prescribe diamorphine, dipipanone, or cocaine for treating addiction but may prescribe these items for treating organic disease or injury
Pharmacist prescriber[1]	• *Non-controlled drugs*: Any medicine provided it is not blacklisted[2] • *Controlled drugs*: Schedule 2, 3, 4, and 5—are not able to prescribe diamorphine, dipipanone, or cocaine for treating addiction but may prescribe these items for treating organic disease or injury	• *Non-controlled drugs*: Any medicine • *Controlled drugs*: Schedule 2, 3, 4, and 5—are not able to prescribe diamorphine, dipipanone, or cocaine for treating addiction but may prescribe these items for treating organic disease or injury

[1]Must have successfully completed the appropriate prescribing training programme.
[2]The blacklist and the Drug Tariff apply in primary care only. The 'blacklist' refers to a range of medicines, such as hypnotics and anxiolytics, that cannot be prescribed by brand name.

5.3 Factors to consider when prescribing a medicine for a patient

When prescribing medication for a patient various legal and clinical aspects need to be considered.

Legal perspectives of prescribing

Many medicines are only available on a prescription and are termed prescription-only medicines (POM). Those who call themselves prescribers need to ensure that they are prescribing within the realms of their professional practice and that is the duty of the professional concerned.

  See Chapter 3 for more about POMs.

All licensed medicines available in the UK have a market authorization (MA) or product licence (PL) granted by the Medicines and Healthcare products Regulatory Agency (MHRA). The terms of the MA define what this medication is clinically indicated for, at what dose, for which group of patients, for what duration of treatment, and so on (MHRA, 2008). All medicines have a Summary of Product Characteristics (SPC), which contains a description of the product and the conditions attached to its use. All prescribers need to ensure that their prescribing patterns fall within the MA of the products that they are suggesting for treatment.

In order for a medicine to gain an MA a series of clinical trials need to take place to prove the effectiveness and safety of the new drug. There are occasionally situations where a prescriber may wish to prescribe a medicine before it has obtained an MA. Such a situation would be termed prescribing an **unlicensed** medicine. As a prescriber you would take full legal responsibility should anything adverse occur to patients while they are taking an unlicensed medicine. This situation differs from prescribing a licensed medicine outside its

FIGURE 5.2 Details of the legal and clinical requirements for a prescription

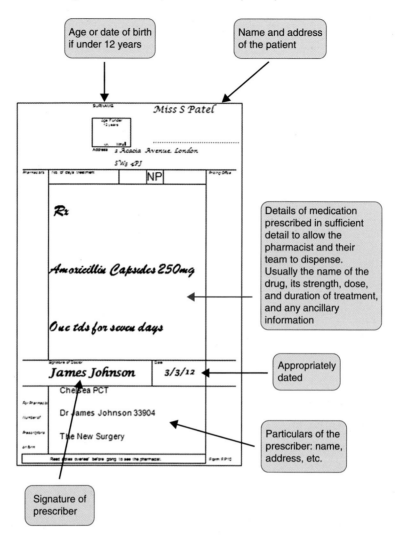

MA, which would be termed off-label prescribing (see Case Study 5.1).

Writing the prescription

In terms of writing the prescription, the prescriber needs to ensure that all of the legal requirements for a prescription are fulfilled. These include:

- Name and address of the patient
- Age or date of birth if under 12 years
- Signature of prescriber
- Dated appropriately
- Particulars of the prescriber:
  - Such particulars as to indicate whether the prescriber is a doctor, dentist, community practitioner, nurse prescriber, nurse independent prescriber, optometrist, pharmacist, European Economic Area (EEA) or Swiss doctor, or an EEA or Swiss dentist
  - Name and address
- Written in indelible ink or computer generated.

More information about prescription writing is contained at the front of the *BNF*, where there are a number of useful subsections. In addition, some medications that are prescribed fall into a category called controlled

Ms Cook is a pharmacist prescriber. She prescribes Depakote® 500 mg tablets to two patients: a 56-year-old man with migraines, as prophylaxis, and a 17-year-old woman with bipolar disorder.

In the Summary of Product Characteristics for Depakote® 500 mg tablets (PL number 04425/0200), Section 4 'Pharmaceutical form', states:

- Regarding therapeutic indications: 'Treatment of manic episode in bipolar disorder when lithium is contraindicated or not tolerated. The continuation of treatment after manic episode could be considered in patients who have responded to Depakote for acute mania.'

- Regarding children and adolescents: 'The safety and efficacy of Depakote for the treatment of manic episodes in bipolar disorder have not been evaluated in patients aged less than 18 years.'

REFLECTION QUESTIONS

1. Both of these cases are examples of **off-label** prescribing. For both patients, explain why this is.

2. Why might a prescriber be more likely to prescribe off-label for children than adults?

3. What reasons might a prescriber give for choosing an off-label medication for their patient?

Answers

1 If a prescriber uses Depakote® for migraine prophylaxis then they would be using it outside its therapeutic indication and so it is 'off-label' or 'off-licence'. The prescriber in this case takes full professional responsibility if anything adverse occurs to the patient. In the case of the 17-year-old the prescribing would be also be called 'off-label' because the prescriber is following the therapeutic indication but prescribing to a patient who is not included in the market authorization. Again, the prescriber takes professional responsibility for this.

2 The General Medical Council supplementary guidance document, *Good practice in prescribing medicines: guidance for doctors*, states: 'Currently pharmaceutical companies do not usually test their medicines on children and, as a consequence, cannot apply to license their medicines for use in the treatment of children. The use of medicines that have been licensed for adults, but not for children, is often necessary in paediatric practice.'

3 If a prescriber chooses an off-label medication they must be satisfied that (1) it is more appropriate for the patient than a licensed alternative and (2) there is sufficient evidence or experience to show its safety and effectiveness.

---

drugs (CD). These are categorized in schedules from 1 to 5, where Schedule 1 are non-prescribable owing to a general lack of therapeutic use. For Schedules 2 and 3, owing to their potential for abuse, there are additional legal requirements when prescribing:

- The dose prescribed needs to be clear and not 'as directed'.

- Treatment length not to exceed 30 days.

- Total quantity needs to be written in both words and figures; for example, 28 and twenty-eight.

- If the medicine is to be given in instalments these need to be specified.

 See Chapter 3 for more in-depth coverage of the legal aspects of medicines.

The prescriber must include a number of practical items necessary for dispensing:

- Name of the drug
- Dose of the drug

- Strength if more than one available
- Dosage form
- Duration of treatment or total quantity required
- Any instructions in addition to those around dosing.

Clinical perspectives of prescribing

The word 'clinical' generally refers to the treatment of patients. There needs to be a general understanding that the patient is at the centre of the disease management and their personal factors should be considered before prescribing. Prescribers should approach this in a stepwise manner; that is, going from the clinician's history taking to physical examinations, objective tests, and then a working diagnosis.

History taking

Taking the patient's medical history is vital to assisting the prescriber's diagnosis. Good communication skills are required to ensure that the patient feels able to talk openly and freely to their prescriber and pharmacist about their current condition, its history, and their feelings and beliefs around health. As part of questioning the patient, their previous medical history (PMH) also needs to be taken into account. Taking an accurate medical history is important to establish anything that may be contributing to or exacerbating the current complaint. Any treatment that the patient has taken for their current complaint, or medication they take for other conditions, needs to be investigated together with any herbal, homeopathic, and traditional ethnic medicines, health supplements, creams, patches, or other forms of treatment. With a clearer picture through a thorough investigation the prescriber is in a position to make a working diagnosis of the current complaint and how this might fit with any other pre-existing medical conditions or pathologies. Finally, before considering prescribing for the current condition, any allergies or ineffective previous treatments need to be investigated.

 See Chapter 7 for more in-depth coverage of patients and factors affecting their health and beliefs around illness.

Physical examination

During discussion with the patient, a number of other areas may need to be investigated to ascertain a working diagnosis. The prescriber may need to perform a physical examination of the patient by using inspection, **palpation**, **percussion**, or **auscultation**. For example, if a patient went to their prescriber complaining of a pain in their chest they would expect the prescriber to discuss this and listen to their heart and lungs using a stethoscope.

Objective tests

The prescriber may also need to conduct a range of objective tests. Some of these can be carried out during the consultation and the results obtained instantaneously. For example, the prescriber may need to measure the patient's blood pressure or may wish to measure the patient's lung function using a peak flow meter. Some tests may be carried out during the consultation but the results may not be known for some time. Samples of blood or other body fluids have to be sent to a laboratory and prescribers may have to delay the start of treatment. Other tests may involve the use of specialized equipment such as magnetic resonance imaging (MRI) scanners, and the patient would be referred to secondary care for the test.

Working diagnosis

The patient's history and the results of the physical examination and objective tests will be put together to help form a working diagnosis. This will help to establish the options for treatment. If treatment is successful then the working diagnosis may be confirmed and if it is not successful then the prescriber may need to re-evaluate their working diagnosis and conduct further testing.

Prescribing decision-making

When considering what the treatment options are, the first decision is likely to be whether to treat or not to treat the patient. In some cases, such as some viral infections, the condition may not require treatment. In such situations the prescriber may need to educate the patient regarding the lack of need for medication other than analgesics for fever and pain relief. In other cases the patient may not wish to receive treatment and that is obviously their choice. It is much better that the prescriber establishes the patient's views regarding treatment at this point rather than prescribing an item that the patient will not take.

Once the prescriber and patient have agreed that a medicine will be used to treat the patient they need to select an appropriate medicine. The decision should be based upon the best available evidence and the term used to describe this is evidence-based medicine. There may also be a national or a local guideline in place that could influence prescribing decisions. Prescribers can deviate from guidelines but they must be prepared to justify why they have done so. A reason for deviation could be because the patient is taking other medicines that interact with the recommended medicine, or that they cannot tolerate it. There may also be a local formulary (list of medicines) in place and prescribers are likely to be expected to prescribe a formulary medicine before a non-formulary medicine.

 See Chapter 8 for a description of evidence-based medicine.

In some cases the medicine with the greatest amount of evidence supporting its use may not be suitable for an individual patient (Box 5.1 gives more information on cautions, contraindications, and interactions). For example, angiotensin-converting enzyme (ACE) inhibitor drugs do not work well in patients from an Afro-Caribbean background, so would not be the first choice. Some drugs may exacerbate certain pre-existing conditions and so should be avoided. A patient who presents with a chest infection may be prescribed an antibiotic and a sympathomimetic such as pseudoephedrine to ease nasal congestion. Nasal congestion is caused by dilated blood vessels, and the vasoconstricting action of pseudoephedrine provides symptomatic relief. Unfortunately, it affects all blood vessels around the body. If the patient were also suffering from hypertension the vasoconstrictor effect would increase their blood pressure, making the medicine unsuitable (contraindicated) for that patient.

When patients take more than one type of drug there is a possibility that the drugs could interact with each other (Box 5.1). It is important to also consider over-the-counter medicines and herbal remedies when considering potential drug interactions. Some interactions are not limited to drugs and could include foods, alcohol, or tobacco. Interactions are usually considered in a negative light but it is important to realize that many interactions are beneficial and some combinations of drugs may be given together deliberately to interact. Some antihypertensive medications are frequently given together to help lower blood pressure to an even greater degree. If drugs work together to enhance the effects this is called a synergistic effect. An example would be an ACE inhibitor and a thiazide diuretic or a calcium-channel blocker used for hypertension. If these drugs were given concomitantly they would cause a bigger than expected drop in blood pressure. Combinations like this are often seen in the pharmacy because the prescriber has taken a consideration of this effect, but should always be confirmed.

KEY POINT

Prescribing should be based upon the best available evidence and should also take the patient's circumstances (medical history, other medicines, and comorbidities) into account.

BOX 5.1

Cautions, contraindications, and drug interactions

The BNF lists cautions and contraindications within the drug monographs.

Cautions

A caution describes a situation where a patient is at greater risk of experiencing harm from the medicine. It could mean that the medicine is less suitable for some patients or that greater monitoring is required.

For example, β-blocking drugs such as propranolol are cautioned in diabetes. It is known that these drugs can interfere with glucose metabolism and that they can mask the symptoms of hypoglycaemia. The risk of harm in patients who are unlikely to suffer hypoglycaemia is relatively low but it would be wise to avoid propranolol in patients who have frequent hypoglycaemic episodes

Contraindications

A contraindication is where the licence states that the medicine should not be used.

For example, propranolol is contraindicated in asthma. β-blocking drugs can precipitate bronchospasm and the consequences of this are potentially very serious so they are contraindicated in patients with a history of bronchospasm.

Drug interactions

The BNF also provides a list of drug interactions. Searching interactions in the BNF is not nearly as straightforward as it sounds. Most but not all drugs are listed by drug class. To determine the class of a particular drug it is sometimes necessary to look at the monograph and work back to the start of the section.

For example, warfarin interactions can be found under the drug class name of coumarins but dipyridamole is listed under its own drug name. In time, experience helps pharmacists to search in the correct place but until that time it is important to search under all the different terms before you can be certain that there is definitely no interaction.

A prescriber may need to issue a prescription before test results come back from the laboratory. For example, a patient who presents with a very chesty cough with coloured (yellow, green, or brown) sputum may have a lower respiratory tract infection. Ideally, a sample of sputum would be sent to the laboratory to confirm which bacteria are involved in the infection in order to determine the most appropriate antibiotic, but, in practice, a broad-spectrum antibiotic such as amoxicillin will probably be prescribed to avoid delaying treatment. Once the test results are back then the patient may need to be prescribed different antibiotic medication if it is found that their infection is resistant to amoxicillin.

When selecting which drug to give to a patient the prescriber also needs to consider:

- Formulation (would the patient prefer a tablet, capsule, slow-release formulation, etc?).

- Duration of treatment.
- Action that the patient needs to take if this treatment does not work.
- Other investigations or referrals to other HCP.
- The ability of the patient to take the medication as intended.
- Side effects of the medication and whether these are tolerable to the patient.
- Adverse drug reactions and how to warn the patient.

If the patient's condition is acute (short-lasting, such as a chest infection) then they will probably only need a short course of treatment to cure the problem. Their prescriber should inform them what to do should the situation not resolve after the course of medication. This message should be reinforced by the pharmacist.

5.4 Chronic or long-term prescribing

If a patient has a chronic or long-term condition then at the first diagnosis they will usually be given a medication in line with national guidelines. They will generally be issued with a prescription for a short period and reviewed frequently until they are stabilized. For conditions such as hypertension or asthma they may be given 1 month's treatment and asked to return to the prescriber to review treatment choice, medication efficacy (is the drug working?), and suitability (is it causing any unacceptable side effects?). Once stabilized on regular treatment the patient will be reviewed less frequently, depending

on their condition. At this stage the medication they receive will be identical each month. This is commonly referred to as repeat prescribing. Patients (or, if arranged, someone acting on their behalf) usually collect their repeat prescriptions from their general practitioner's (GP) surgery or the pharmacy. Repeat supplies of the medicine can be formally organized in conjunction with a community pharmacist via the repeat dispensing scheme. Under this scheme the GP issues a prescription that has 6 months' worth of repeats, which are kept at the pharmacy and dispensed one month at a time.

5.5 Ethical perspectives of prescribing

The patient's welfare is the primary concern of all HCPs and codes of ethics for most professions will include a statement to that end. Ensuring patient safety is therefore paramount. Unfortunately, no medicine is ever without risk of adverse effects. The role of the

prescriber and pharmacist in all situations is to weigh up the balance of the benefits of prescribing versus the potential risks of treatment. For example, the drug thalidomide was used in the 1960s to treat morning sickness in pregnant women. Although it worked very well for its indicated condition it also had adverse effects in the unborn fetus, causing malformed or unformed limbs; it was teratogenic. Therefore, the risk–benefit ratio here was too high. This led to the formation in 1963 of the Committee on Safety of Medicines (CSM), which is now part of the MHRA. Thalidomide is now used to help slow the progression of some cancers such as multiple myeloma, and as long as the patient does not become pregnant it will not affect them as previously described.

 See Chapter 3 in *Pharmaceutical Chemistry* within this series for more information on the effect of stereochemistry on drug action.

When patients visit their prescriber they might expect that they will receive a prescription to cure or treat their medical condition. Sometimes, it may be in the best interests of the patient or the public at large not to prescribe a medicine. However, the prescriber is in a difficult ethical situation owing to this expectation. For example, research has shown that the majority of cases of otitis media (middle-ear infection) in children are viral in origin. Therefore, antibiotics will not work and could contribute to the rise of resistant strains of bacteria. Also, side effects experienced while taking antibiotics are common and include nausea, vomiting, and diarrhoea. While the parent may want an antibiotic as their child is in pain and crying, the best option may be to prescribe not antibiotics but simple analgesics. As a middle ground to help both the patient and prescriber, a post-dated prescription may be given to the parent to be presented to the pharmacy in 2 days' time if the child is no better.

 See Chapter 1 and Chapter 3 for more on professionalism and ethical considerations.

5.6 Economic perspectives of prescribing

91

Prescribers must consider the cost of the items they prescribe. There is the cost of the medicine itself and someone, or some organization, must pay this cost. NHS costs are ultimately met by the taxpayer, while private prescription costs are met by an insurance company, an employer, or the patients themselves. Many prescribers are allocated a budget for prescribing. With a cash-limited budget there may be a dilemma for prescribers around prescribing the optimum therapy for the patient and staying within budget (see Case Study 5.2).

In the UK there is a growing debate about NHS charges for prescriptions. In Wales, Scotland, and Northern Ireland patients do not pay a fee for their NHS prescription. In England, the fee paid per prescription item has grown steadily over the years and is a contribution to the actual cost of the drugs prescribed. However, it is estimated that about 90% of items dispensed to patients in England are exempt from prescription charges anyway.

 See Chapter 2 and Chapter 8 for more information on prescription charges and how they should be considered.

 See Chapter 8 for more in-depth coverage of economic perspectives.

5.7 Factors to consider when dispensing a prescription for a patient

Once the prescription has been written and presented to the pharmacy a particular journey is taken through the dispensary that leads to the medicine being ready to be supplied to the patient. A pharmacist must ensure

CASE STUDY 5.2

John visits his pharmacist prescriber, Mr Parker, as he has the symptoms of moderate depression. Mr Parker agrees that an antidepressant medication might be beneficial to John, so he consults his *BNF*. There are a number of medications that would be suitable for prescribing and the *BNF* notes 'there is little to choose between the different classes of drugs in terms of efficacy'.

He looks at the costs of two potential medicines:

- Amitriptyline 100 mg per day = £0.92 for 14 days (0.07p per day)

- Escitalopram 10 mg per day = £14.91 for 28 days (0.53p per day)

Despite the fact that escitalopram 10 mg is more expensive, Mr Parker decides to prescribe it for John.

REFLECTION QUESTION

Besides cost, what other factors would Mr Parker have considered before making his choice?

Answer

Section 5.3 covers what factors to consider when prescribing a medicine for a patient. Examples include whether a medicine is licensed to treat the patient's condition, whether the patient is likely to take the medication in the form available, and whether they are likely to have any adverse side effects.

In this case, Mr Parker is likely to have selected escitalopram over amitriptyline because escitalopram is a selective serotonin-reuptake inhibitor (SSRI). SSRIs are recommended as first-line treatment for depression as they are better tolerated and safer in overdose.

that all legal, clinical, and ethical checks have been completed and that the medicine is appropriate and safe for the patient. The order in which these checks occur does not matter, provided they happen before the medication is issued to the patient. Once checks have taken place then the actual dispensing of the prescription can occur. The final check is an accuracy check, which involves comparing the dispensed item with the prescription. This is obviously a vital step as errors at this point can lead to patient harm. All processes involving humans are liable to result in errors at some point and pharmacy staff must be vigilant to minimize this risk. Some pharmacies employ an accredited checking technician (ACT) who has passed an accuracy checking assessment and can check the final item is safe for the patient. Where there is no ACT the pharmacist has the responsibility for the final check.

Standard operating procedures

In order to be safe and consistent, pharmacies have been required to have **standard operating procedures (SOPs)** for dispensing since 1 January 2005. SOPs are structured instructions stating what is to be done and by whom. The SOP must specify the activities covered, the objective of the SOP, who is responsible, what the procedure is, and describe how the procedure will be audited.

Each SOP should consist of two parts. First, there should be an outline or summary that defines the process or procedure included in the SOP. Second would be a detailed description of the process or stages to be completed. This would also include which member of staff was responsible and any other important information, together with a date to review the SOP. While standard templates can be obtained from various organizations such as the National Pharmaceutical Association and Royal Pharmaceutical Society, each SOP has to be tailored to the pharmacy where it will operate.

KEY POINT

It is necessary to have a standard operating procedure in place that makes it clear who is responsible for dispensing medicines.

 See Chapter 2 for more in-depth coverage of clinical governance and the organization of health care.

Legal perspectives of prescription handling

As described in Section 5.3, the prescriber has a duty to ensure that the prescription is written legally and any omissions on the part of the prescriber will need to be clarified and amended.

Some prescriptions may require alteration because they either do not contain all the information needed for dispensing or they contain incorrect information. Some changes to prescriptions, such as the patient's date of birth, could be clarified by talking to the parent or patient; an endorsement of 'PNC' or 'prescriber not contacted' would then be written on the prescription by the pharmacist. Other aspects which are a legal requirement, such as the prescriber's signature, cannot be completed by the dispensing pharmacist and the document is not valid without this. If this occurs, the pharmacist should arrange to have the prescription signed before dispensing the item. Generally, the legal items are contained in the area around the middle body of the prescription.

Clinical perspectives of prescription handling

The pharmacist who dispenses generally performs the final safety check, and it is vital that they clinically check the prescription to ensure that the medication is safe and appropriate for the patient. The pharmacist checks the main body of the prescription (indicated with a red arrow in Figure 5.2) to ensure that the medication is suitable for that patient. If the patient has a patient medication record (PMR) then this can be checked to ensure consistency for repeat prescriptions of earlier medication. If this patient has been prescribed a new medication, either for their chronic condition or something else, then the pharmacist checks that it is compatible with the patient's regular medication (see Box 5.2). Also, the prescription will be checked clinically to confirm that the medication is appropriate for the condition that the patient is suffering from at the prescribed dose, dose frequency, and duration of treatment.

If the patient is not known to that pharmacy then the pharmacist will probably need to check some

BOX 5.2

Clinical checks

Clinical checks to go through before prescribing a medication to a patient:

- Is it a new therapy?
    - Is the medication indicated?
    - Is it appropriate and recommended? (evidence-based medicine or local guidelines)
    - Is the formulation appropriate?
- Are there any cautions?
- Are there any contraindications?
- Is the dose appropriate?
- Are there any interactions with an existing drug or disease?
- Is the patient allergic to the medicine or its components?
- Is the duration appropriate?

information with the patient to ensure they have a clear understanding of the prescription before them. Should any of this information be missing or need clarification then the pharmacist will call the prescriber to confirm the situation. In this case, the pharmacist endorses the prescription with 'PC' or prescriber contacted. Some pharmacies are connected electronically to GP surgeries, so patient records are accessible, but the vast majority of pharmacies are not, hence the need to telephone.

 See Chapter 8 for more in-depth coverage of pharmaceutical care.

SELF CHECK 5.1

James Vickers (age 32 years) presents a prescription for 15 diclofenac 25 mg tablets, one to be taken three times a day. You see from his records that he has been taking venlafaxine 75 mg XL, one capsule per day, for the last 4 months. What would you do?

Ethical perspectives of prescription handling

Having completed a 4-year programme of study to become a pharmacist, it is the pharmacist's duty, according to the General Pharmaceutical Council's (GPhC) *Standards of Conduct, Ethics and Performance* to 'make patients your first concern'. This means that if you find that there is a problem, in this case on the prescription, you have a duty of care to the patient to resolve this. This is not just about ensuring that no harm is caused to the patient but about proactively making certain that the safest, most effective treatment is given. A problem on a prescription could be a less than optimal dose, which will not necessarily cause harm but is not giving the patient the best treatment either. The pharmacist still has a duty of care to intervene in this case.

It may mean, for example, that you discuss the prescription with the patient, call the prescriber to discuss the situation, or visit them in their practice. Whatever the situation, it is the pharmacist's responsibility to ensure that all of the issues are resolved before issuing the medication to the patient. Sometimes these situations become difficult to handle because the patient or prescriber may put pressure on the pharmacist to follow their wishes. However, as professionals, pharmacists are autonomous, meaning that they need to follow their own professional judgement and not be influenced by others where patients' care and safety could be at risk. If a pharmacist issues a medicine to a patient and this subsequently causes harm to the patient then both the pharmacist and prescriber would be held liable in law. Therefore, when ethical dilemmas occur it is important to consider the risks and benefits of giving the medication compared with the risks and benefits of not giving the medication. In practice, there are various models or SOPs on how to handle ethical dilemmas. They usually entail seeking further information, discussing the situation with all parties involved, and working out all the possible options together with the consequences of each one. This then leads to making a choice of one of these options together with keeping records of the event and outcome. The GPhC's website contains a number of case studies that you could review.

> **KEY POINT**
>
> The pharmacist is the final check before the patient takes the medicine and it is the pharmacist's duty to ensure that all issues are resolved prior to the patient receiving the medicine.

 See Chapter 1 for more in-depth coverage of professionalism and Chapter 3 for more on ethical perspectives.

5.8 Preparing the medicine

Once all legal, clinical, and ethical perspectives have been reviewed then the item may be labelled and dispensed ready for issuing to the patient.

Labelling of prescribed medicines

Every item on a prescription, by law, needs to be labelled in accordance with the directions of the prescriber. The purpose of the label is to enable the patient to take their medication safely and obtain the maximum benefit from treatment. The label usually follows a standard format seen across all pharmacies, except for patients with any special requirements. For example, a patient who is partially sighted may need a large print or Braille label. Figure 5.3 shows what the label should include.

All of the items on the label can be double checked with the use of the *BNF*. This helps the pharmacist confirm the usual dose, forms, and strengths of the medication being prescribed. The *BNF* recommends the addition of cautionary and advisory labels to provide additional information for the patient. These

FIGURE 5.3   General requirements for labelling dispensed medicines for human use

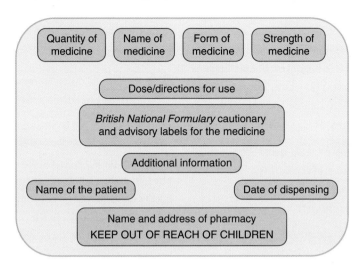

cautionary and advisory labels are additional to the standard additional labels such as: 'shake the bottle' or 'for external use only'. They are intended to provide advice on how the medicine should be used, such as: 'dissolve this medicine under your tongue' or to warn the patient, such as: 'This medicine may make you sleepy. If this happens do not drive or use tools or machines.' Pharmacists must use their judgement when deciding which cautionary and advisory labels to use because some may be less relevant; for example, 'avoid alcohol' in medicines for use in young children. The *BNF* lists all of the cautionary and advisory labels for dispensed medicines.

SELF CHECK 5.2

What advisory or cautionary labels would you place of the following: (a) 56 propranolol 80 mg MR capsules for Rachel Vickers, aged 31; (b) azithromycin capsules for Dilip Patel, aged 55; (c) 14 doxycycline 100 mg capsules for Ravi Patel; (d) 100 ml chlorphenamine syrup for Maya Vickers, aged 3.

Figure 5.4 shows what the label would look like for the medication prescribed in Figure 5.2. By labelling this item carefully and precisely, and counselling the patient appropriate to their level of understanding, Miss Patel can now go home and refer to the label for instructions on how to take her medicine. Further, where a medicine is supplied it should be accompanied

FIGURE 5.4   Example of a label that would be associated with the prescription in Figure 5.2

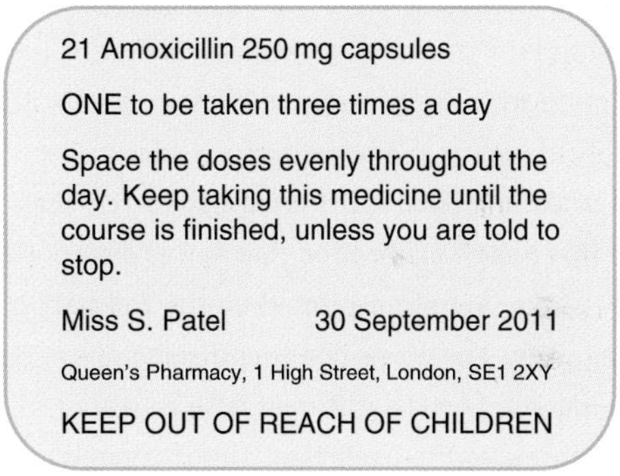

> 21 Amoxicillin 250 mg capsules
>
> ONE to be taken three times a day
>
> Space the doses evenly throughout the day. Keep taking this medicine until the course is finished, unless you are told to stop.
>
> Miss S. Patel   30 September 2011
>
> Queen's Pharmacy, 1 High Street, London, SE1 2XY
>
> KEEP OUT OF REACH OF CHILDREN

by a Patient Information Leaflet (PIL). This contains additional information about the product that has been dispensed, such as side effects, what to do in the case of missing a dose, and so on. It is important to also remember the personal touch; counselling the patient about their medication personally will lead to a better understanding of their treatment and options. For example, the patient may have difficulty reading or understanding the PIL. Counselling can help to reinforce important points or help to allay fears or concerns. This will be covered in more detail in Section 5.7.

In certain cases items will have a particular expiry date that needs to be communicated to the patient. For example, any sterile products (such as eye drops) will only last for 28 days once opened. Most regular medicines such as tablets have a much longer expiry date of a few years so it is important that the pharmacy regularly checks that their stock is in date and safe for patients to take. When a medicine has a short expiry date then it is vital that the patient is informed to use this medicine before it expires. If a medicine is used after its expiry date it may have lost potency or it may have become contaminated and cause harm to the patient.

 See Chapter 7 for more in-depth coverage of patients and factors affecting their health and beliefs around illness.

Preparation of standard prescribed medicines

Most medicines supplied in pharmacies are in the form of single-use or original packs. These are packs of medicines that will last the patient for 1 month or one standard course of treatment. Often, solid oral dosage forms are packaged in blister packs with foil and plastic coating. A benefit of calendar packs is that they make it easier for the patient to see that they have taken their medication that day as days of week/times of day are often printed on the foil part of the blister pack. The corresponding disadvantage is that if the patient needs a different dose to standard then this information is irrelevant. Unfortunately, not all manufacturers can agree on the number of days in a month. While the calendar has 28-, 29-, 30-, and 31-day months, in pharmacy it is usual to have 28- or 30-day calendar packs.

Some medicines, such as antibiotic syrups for children or adults with difficulty swallowing tablets, come into the pharmacy as dry powder or granules to be reconstituted with water. Such medicines are not supplied already reconstituted because the drug will hydrolyse in an aqueous environment and so is not stable pharmaceutically. The pharmaceutical manufacturer therefore prepares a specific quantity of dry powder or granules in a bottle, which gives a longer shelf life. The pharmacist or one of their staff then reads from the side of the bottle for the amount of water required for reconstitution. This bottle needs some 'additional information' to be put on the label so that the patient has the greatest benefit; in this case:

'shake the bottle'. Mixtures will often settle on standing, so to ensure the dose in each 5 ml spoonful is the same the bottle needs to be shaken to redisperse any sediment.

 See Chapter 10 of *Pharmaceutics* within this series for more information about disperse systems.

While calendar packs and single-course liquids are useful for patients, liquid medicines are often supplied in bulk containers for decanting into smaller bottles for dispensing. For example, paracetamol syrup 120 mg/5 ml could be in the dispensary in 2-litre bottles. Careful pouring is required because this liquid is very viscous.

When working in the pharmacy you may come across medication that could be harmful to you or other staff working in that area. For example, methotrexate is a cytotoxic medication and can cause immunosuppression. It is used to treat severe rheumatic disease, cancer, and inflammatory bowel disease, among other things. Mostly it is packaged in calendar packs, but sometimes it will be supplied to the pharmacy in larger containers. There should be a SOP available that covers using gloves and having designated tablet-counting equipment for this purpose only in order to minimize the risk to the staff handling the medicine.

Preparation of extemporaneously dispensed items

Historically, pharmacy played an important role in manufacturing small quantities of medication for specific patients following the instructions from the prescriber. Using a formula (or recipe), various techniques for mixing ingredients effectively was followed leading to the production of a pharmaceutically consistent and elegant product. These products were termed 'extemporaneously prepared' and were commonplace in the pharmacy. The term extemporaneously dispensed is derived from dispensing without previous preparation (that is, they are made to order) as opposed to most other items, which are manufactured elsewhere in advance. It has been defined as 'the manipulation by pharmacists of various drug and chemical ingredients using traditional compounding techniques to produce suitable medicines when no commercial form is available'. In more recent times, owing to the general lack of aseptic equipment in the pharmacy and the impact of legislation such as Control of Substances Hazardous to Health (COSHH) 1994 (and amendments), community pharmacy tends to send off such prescribed items for special manufacture. These items are called 'specials' and the units that make them must have the appropriate MHRA licence. They are often located in large hospitals or are part of chain of community pharmacies.

In the past, the main types of item that were made up by the pharmacy were special recipes for products that maybe a hospital consultant had ordered. For example, in dermatology, a non-standard strength of cream; in ophthalmology, a special formulation of sterile eye drops etc. The manufacture of such items is beyond the remit of this book.

 See the *Pharmaceutics* volume for a more detailed discussion.

5.9 Accuracy checking of the dispensed item

After a pharmacist has conducted the clinical and legal checks on the prescription, and the item has been prepared and labelled, the final step in the process is the accuracy check. At this stage the item and labels will be checked for accuracy and similarity. Here, the pharmacist or ACT is double checking all aspects of the product in front of them. Steps involved in the process will include:

- Dispensed drug as stated on the prescription.
- Correct strength as stated on the prescription.
- Correct dose on the label and prescription.
- Correct form as stated on the prescription.
- Correct quantity dispensed and as stated on the prescription.
- Expiry date.
- Package contains a PIL.

Once the final accuracy check has been completed the dispensed medicine is put into a bag and closed ready to be issued to the patient with any instructions for safe and effective use.

5.10 Giving the medicine to the patient

Patient counselling, advice, and information

Using medicines appropriately and safely is not always straightforward. Good communication skills are vital to ensure that the messages concerning medicine usage that you need to get across to the patient are received and understood. It is also important that communication is two-way, so that the patient is able to voice any concerns or ask any questions.

While the label produced for the medication contains all the legal requirements, it is important that the pharmacist or delegated member of staff talks to all patients about their medicines. Talking to the patient about their medicines can alleviate any worries, anxieties, or fears, and allows a trusting relationship to develop. For the prescription in Figure 5.2 you could say something to the patient such as:

Miss Patel, you have been given some antibiotic capsules for your infection. You need to take one capsule every

8 hours and you must take them until the packet is finished, even if you feel better. This means that the medicine will kill all of the bugs causing you to feel ill in the first place. Sometimes they might make you feel a little sick, but you can take these with food so that should help. Don't worry if you forget a dose, just take one as soon as you remember. Do you have any questions?

Patients will often have more questions about their medicines than you anticipate and it is important to be prepared to answer them. There will be times when you do not know the answer to questions you are asked. When the patient asks you a question you cannot answer it is important that you remain confident in front of them and explain that you need to check the answer. Examples of the type of question that a patient may ask include the following:

- Do I take my medicine before or after food?
- What happens if my condition does not get better?
- What are the side effects of this medicine?
- Can I drink alcohol with this medicine?
- What if I miss a dose?
- What if I take too many?
- Will it interact with any of my other medicines?

> **KEY POINT**
>
> It is vital to be able to communicate effectively with the patient and, where possible, to prepare for each patient consultation.

 See Chapter 7 for more in-depth coverage of patient beliefs.

Ongoing monitoring and review

If the patient is taking their medication for a long-term chronic condition such as hypertension then it is good practice to discuss with the patient any ongoing monitoring or review that needs to take place. For example, this patient may need to visit their prescriber every year for their annual check-up. In addition, pharmacies in England are able to offer a Medicines Use Review for patients.

In England, the New Medicines Service has recently been introduced. Under the terms of this service pharmacists arrange follow-up meetings for patients who have been prescribed a new medicine for asthma, chronic obstructive pulmonary disease, type 2 diabetes, or hypertension, or who have received anticoagulant or antiplatelet therapy. The aim of the service is to provide support, encouragement, and lifestyle advice, which will hopefully lead to improved adherence and reduced waste (see Box 5.3).

 See Chapter 8 for more in-depth coverage of pharmaceutical care.

Adherence and compliance are useful terms when they are used in academic studies to describe a patient's behaviour but they are less useful when considering how to address differences in the views of the prescriber and the patient. Adherence often refers to a retrospective discussion asking the patient how they followed their instructions. Conversely, compliance suggests that the patient must follow the instructions in an almost paternalistic manner. The decision regarding whether to take a medicine or not should be one that is reached by both the prescriber and patient. The word **concordance** has been used to describe developing a shared agenda and agreeing a plan for medicine taking.

 See Chapter 7 for more in-depth coverage of patient beliefs.

> **KEY POINT**
>
> Non-adherence can be intentional or unintentional. It is important to explore the patient's views regarding medicine use in order to determine how best to support the patient.

Record keeping

It is a legal requirement that the pharmacy keeps records of certain types of prescription items that it dispenses. Prescriptions for many controlled drugs need to be recorded in the controlled drugs register, and private prescriptions for POMs need to be recorded in the private prescription register. Prescription records must be stored in the pharmacy

BOX 5.3

Do patients take their medication?

Several studies have reported that relatively high proportions (30–50%) of patients do not take their medication after it has been dispensed. Each year many patients or their carers return unused medicines to community pharmacies for disposal. It is clear that not taking medicine represents a waste of resources because the NHS has to pay for the medicines to be dispensed in the first place and then pay the costs for disposal.

The terms 'adherence' and 'compliance' have been used to describe how closely a patient's behaviour coincides with the directions of the prescription. If a prescription states take one tablet three times a day for five days and the patient does not follow these directions that would be an example of non-adherence. Non-adherence can occur when a patient takes too much or too little of their medicine, and can be intentional or unintentional.

Non-adherence can be intentional when a patient deliberately decides not to take their medicine. Some patients have an inherent dislike of medicines, some feel that medicines interfere with the body's natural balance, and some believe that they can lead to addiction. Others may have a temporary aversion to medicines triggered

perhaps by something on the news or in a magazine about their medicine and they have decided, after reading this, to stop taking it. Perhaps a patient who was prescribed the antibacterial metronidazole may refuse to take it as they cannot drink alcohol with it. It is not the pharmacist's role to persuade the patient to take their medication but to assist the patient and inform them regarding the risks and benefits of their medication in a manner that they can understand, to allow them to make an informed decision.

Unintentional non-adherence can occur when a patient is unable to take their medication or when they forget to take the medicine. Pharmacy can help by advising on medicine use and changing formulation, or by supplying special boxes (adherence aids). If patients have several medicines to take each day these can help them to remember but it should be noted that patients may have to pay a fee for this. The boxes are often divided into days of the week if the patient only takes medicines once a day. For dosing more than once-daily systems are available that can accommodate any combination, commonly up to four times a day. Examples of systems are shown in Figure 5.5.

FIGURE 5.5 **Aids for patient adherence. A patient's medication can be organized for (a) once-daily dosing (b) four times a day dosing.**
Source: (a) This file is licensed under the Creative Commons Attribution-Share Alike 3.0 Unported license. Copyright: Dvortygirl. (b) Photographer: Corbis.

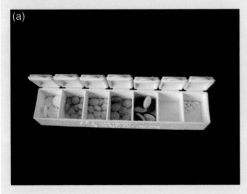
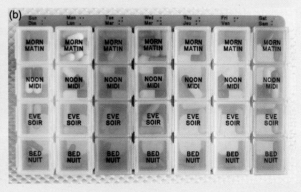

for a minimum of 2 years after the last date of entry in the register.

 See Chapter 3 for a description of the legal categories of medicines.

Final destination of prescriptions

From the perspective of pharmacy, when a prescription is presented by a patient the pharmacy has a duty to supply the medicine with reasonable promptness.

After the medication has been supplied to the patient, NHS prescriptions will be endorsed within the pharmacy to make it clear exactly what was supplied and then filed together with all the others that have been presented that month. They are then bundled together and sent to the appropriate organization, where prescription details are processed and the reimbursement due to the pharmacy is calculated. The reimbursement includes the cost of drugs supplied, an allowance for the container that it was dispensed in, and the fee for dispensing.

There are separate organizations for each part of the UK. In England, prescriptions are sent to NHS Business Service Authority (NHSBSA) Prescriptions Services; in Wales they are sent to Prescribing Services, Shared Services Partnership; in Scotland they are sent to Practitioner Services Pharmacy; and in Northern Ireland they are sent to Business Services Organization.

CHAPTER SUMMARY

➤ This chapter explored the process involved from a patient presenting to their prescriber with a medical condition to the issuing of the prescription to the patient for subsequent use.

➤ There are two types of prescriber. An independent prescriber is responsible for diagnosis and prescribing, whereas a supplementary prescriber is not responsible for diagnosis and must prescribe in accordance with a clinical management plan.

➤ Clinical, legal, and ethical perspectives must be addressed during prescribing and dispensing.

➤ From the many steps in the process it can be seen that errors could be inadvertently introduced, so standard operating procedures (SOP) are required.

➤ Non-adherence can be intentional or unintentional.

➤ Putting the patient at the centre of this process, using legal, ethical, and clinical concepts, means that at all times the target of care is in clear focus.

➤ A patient's medication-taking motivation must be explored to achieve concordance.

FURTHER READING

There are a range of prescription types that may be issued by prescribers working in the community or hospital and there are differences between the different parts of the UK. Further information on the different types of prescription forms is available from:

England: NHS Business Service Authority (NHSBSA). Prescription services. <http://www.nhsbsa.nhs.uk/Prescription Services.aspx>.

Wales: NHS Wales. Shared Services Partnership. Primary care services. <http://www.wales.nhs.uk/sites3/home.cfm?orgid=428>.

Scotland: NHS Scotland. Practitioner Services. Pharmacy services. <http://www.psd.scot.nhs.uk/professionals/pharmacy/pharmacy-services.html>.

Northern Ireland: Health and Social Care in Northern Ireland. Business Services Organisation. <http://www.hscbusiness.hscni.net/services/1944.htm>.

Royal Pharmaceutical Society. *Medicines, Ethics and Practice: A Guide for Pharmacists and Pharmacy Technicians*. 36th edn. Pharmaceutical Press, 2012.

Available as a free download for pharmacy undergraduates when joining the Royal Pharmaceutical Society as a student member.

National Institute for Health and Clinical Excellence. *Medicines Adherence: Involving Patients in Decisions About Prescribed Medicines and Supporting Adherence* Clinical Guideline 76. NICE, 2009. <http://www.nice.org.uk/nicemedia/live/11766/43042/43042.pdf>.

Interaction with other health care professionals and patients

LESLEY DIACK

Health and social care delivery is becoming more and more complex and involves an increasing number of health and social care professionals. Several inquiries in the last decade, including the inquiry into children's heart surgery at the Bristol Royal Infirmary and the tragic death of Victoria Climbié have highlighted what can go wrong when there is ineffective collaboration between health care professionals. High-profile failures in health care feature prominently in the media, creating negative perceptions not only of health care professionals but also of their teamworking skills. These inquiries have identified and demonstrated the need to increase and expand interprofessional education. Thus health professionals can develop collaborative work practices from their undergraduate studies onwards and can help to increase communication in multidisciplinary teams. The importance of interprofessional education has been recognized by the General Pharmaceutical Council and is especially identified in its accreditation of schools of pharmacy documentation.

Learning objectives

Having read this chapter you are expected to be able to:

➤ Understand the roles of the different health and social care professionals.

➤ Describe the origins of interprofessional working.

➤ List the attributes of interdisciplinary teamworking and discuss professional socialization within teams.

➤ Relate the development of interprofessional education and working.

➤ Review the impact of current initiatives on interprofessional working and on health and social care systems.

➤ Describe the expectations that are placed on health and social care teams.

➤ Describe the different professional and regulatory bodies that have an impact on interprofessional working.

➤ Discuss the relationship between the health care professional and the patient.

6.1 The interprofessional team

Health care is provided by a large number of different health and social care professionals. For example, patients admitted to hospital are cared for by a health and social care team that may include doctors, nurses, paramedics, physiotherapists, radiographers, dieticians, occupational therapists, social workers, and psychologists. Similarly, in the community, patients are treated by a large number of health and social care professionals. Pharmacists are key members of these health and social care teams.

The development of an interprofessional or multidisciplinary team requires two things:

1. The development of the individual as a professional, with all the knowledge and understanding that encompasses.
2. An appreciation of the other professions and their strengths and limitations.

By understanding who you are as a professional and where your skills fit in with the people you work alongside, you are supporting the development of a good team. It is important to appreciate your colleagues and their skills, and also to be aware of your own limitations. Key to all of this is effective and efficient communication.

Reflecting the importance of good interprofessional working is Standard 5.5 in the General Pharmaceutical Council's 2011 document *Future Pharmacists: Standards for the Initial Education and Training of Pharmacists*. It states: 'The MPharm degree curriculum must include practical experience of working with patients, carers, and other health care professionals.'

Box 6.1 outlines a few high-profile cases. These cases highlight issues resulting from a lack of teamwork and a lack of knowledge of other professionals' roles and responsibilities, all reinforced by a basic lack of communication. The benefits of interprofessional working are paramount to the improved care of a patient or client. Also, there will be increased job satisfaction for all concerned with a 'job well done'.

KEY POINT

For interprofessional working to occur individuals must have all the knowledge and skills required for their role and must understand the roles of the people they are working with.

BOX 6.1

The need for multidisciplinary or interprofessional teams

In 1998 a public inquiry was established looking into the higher than average number of deaths of children from open heart surgery at Bristol Royal Infirmary. The report found: 'Many failed to communicate with each other, and to work together effectively for the interests of their patients. There was a lack of leadership, and of teamwork.'

In 2000 in London, Victoria Climbié, an 8-year-old girl from the Ivory Coast, was tortured and murdered by her guardians, one of whom was her great-aunt. Her death led to a public inquiry and produced major changes in child protection policies in England, including the 'Every Child Matters' initiative. The Secretary of State for Health at the time, Alan Millburn, is quoted as saying about the case: 'This was not a failing on the part of one service; it was a failing on the part of every service.'

On 18 October 2001, 11-week-old Caleb Alexander Ness was admitted to the Royal Hospital for Sick Children in Edinburgh and pronounced dead. It was immediately suspected that the baby had been the victim of non-accidental injury and his father was subsequently found guilty of culpable homicide. In 2003 the inquiry into the death of Caleb Ness found a number of problems with the health and social care professionals responsible for his care. It was discovered that 'there was a tendency among professionals in all agencies to make assumptions about the knowledge, training and actions of others.'

SELF CHECK 6.1

What is a multidisciplinary team?

SELF CHECK 6.2

Who was Victoria Climbié? Describe how her case has had an impact on child protection policies and how interprofessional teams work together.

6.2 Health and social care professionals: roles and responsibilities

The roles and responsibilities of the health and social care professionals you are most likely to work with are summarized in this section. It is not a complete list, but provides a basic framework and knowledge necessary to any pharmacist. Each of the professions listed does not work in isolation but as part of a team. Many also have specific support workers who are trained to work in conjunction with them.

 See Chapter 2 for more information on the organization of health care in the UK.

Dentist

A dentist is a person who provides preventive and restorative treatments for your teeth and mouth. They have a number of public health roles, helping to develop good oral hygiene and care. Their main concerns are with tooth decay and gum disease, both of which can be symptomatic of other longer-term conditions such as diabetes and heart disease. Dentists are able to prescribe medications to help treat patients. They are helped by a range of auxiliary workers, including dental hygienists, technicians, and nurses. They can work in the National Health Service (NHS) and/or private practice as well as in hospitals, schools, specialist care, and academia. Dentists and pharmacists work together in hospitals. Pharmacists may recommend clients visit a dentist if they have problems with mouth ulcers or other oral ailments.

In the UK, training is for a minimum of 4 or 5 years at university and then further on-the-job training, which is of differing lengths. Since January 2002 continuing professional development (CPD) has been mandatory. All dentists must register with the General Dental Council in order to practise.

Diagnostic radiographer

A diagnostic radiographer uses X-ray technology and a range of specialist imaging equipment to help in the detection, monitoring, and treatment of a patient's illness/injury. Their role has been increasing in recent years to include image interpretation, prescribing of medications, and patient treatment. Radiographers work with patients from across the health service and may work within a variety of environments, which include:

- Accident and emergency departments
- Contrast radiography (examinations to visualize the gastrointestinal and urinary systems)
- Intensive care units
- Operating theatres.

It is seldom that a pharmacist and a diagnostic radiographer will be working together solely on the care of a patient; however, they could often be part of a multidisciplinary team. Training to become a radiographer involves 3 or 4 years at university. Their regulatory body is the Health Professions Council (HPC).

Dietician

Registered dieticians are the only qualified health professionals who assess, diagnose, and treat diet and nutrition problems at both an individual and wider public health level. They develop practical guidance to help individuals make appropriate lifestyle and food decisions, using public health and scientific research on food, health, and disease. They usually work as part of a team caring for people in hospital or in the community. For the NHS, they advise those who need a modified or special diet, such as people with a food allergy or diabetes. Community dieticians are involved in health promotion, public health, and clinical work. Pharmacists and dieticians are both involved in medicines management when nutrition is an important part of the care; for example, advising on food that could affect medicines or on food supplements.

The training is a 4-year undergraduate course at university, which includes a number of long placements, or a 2-year postgraduate course. Their regulatory body is the HPC.

Medical doctor

The role of a doctor is to diagnose and manage a patient's medical condition(s). It is also to protect and promote the health of patients and the public. To establish a diagnosis a medical history must be taken, clinical examinations performed, and relevant investigations carried out. A doctor may be involved in all or part of this process. Management of a condition may include the prescribing of a medication or medications, carrying out practical procedures, ongoing follow-up and tests, and/or referring a patient to other medical specialists or other health care professionals.

In the UK, a doctor has to complete 5 years of undergraduate training and a further year in practice prior to becoming fully registered with the General Medical Council (GMC). All doctors must be registered with the GMC to be able to practise. The GMC produces guidance on the duties of a doctor, which is laid out in the publication *Good Medical Practice*.

Having completed general training, a doctor can choose to specialize. In the community doctors work as general practitioners (GPs). The role of the GP is that of a 'family doctor', who treats the patient for a range of illnesses from acute to chronic, from minor to major but will also refer a patient to a specialist if necessary. GPs have a role to play in health education

and prevention. In hospital there are a number of different medical and surgical specialties, including obstetrics and gynaecology, anaesthetics, the diagnostic specialties (for example, radiology, pathology, microbiology), and psychiatry. Having specialized, doctors will train for a number of years and complete specialist exams before being eligible to apply for a general practitioner or hospital consultant position. Within a hospital there are a number of career positions for a doctor:

- *Foundation doctor*: a newly qualified UK medical graduate on a two-year training period.
- *Specialist or GP trainee*: a doctor who is training for either general practice or a specialty. The length and nature of the training will depend upon the career area/specialty in which the doctor wishes to work.
- *Consultant*: a doctor who is fully trained in a particular specialty area and has overall responsibility for the clinical care of patients. Most consultants work in hospitals in multidisciplinary teams that will include pharmacists, nurses, and other health care professionals as well as other doctors. Consultants are responsible for the education and supervision of junior doctors in their team.

Pharmacists and doctors work closely together in all sectors, in any area of medicines management. Independent prescribing pharmacists will work more closely with a doctor as they take on the role of primary prescriber for patients with long-term conditions.

Midwife

A midwife is the main contact for a woman during normal pregnancy, throughout childbirth, and for a short period after the baby is born. A midwife undertakes clinical examinations and provides health, childbirth, and parenthood education. Midwives work in the community and/or in hospitals. Training to be a midwife usually takes a minimum of 3 years at university, unless already registered with the Nursing and Midwifery Council (NMC) as a nurse, in which case the training would be reduced to

18 months. Half of midwifery training is based in clinical practice, with direct contact with women, their babies, and their families. Midwives work as part of a multidisciplinary team with doctors, nurses, and pharmacists.

Nurse

Nurses are involved in assessing, planning, providing, and evaluating care. Nursing care covers the continuum of life, including death and caring for the bereaved. Nurses are concerned with health improvement, not just sickness and disease. In current health care settings nurses' roles are increasingly autonomous and diverse.

Nurses may work in a variety of settings, including NHS and private hospitals, nursing homes, walk-in health centres, clinics, prisons, schools, and industry. Within a primary care setting, they may be practice nurses within a GP practice, health visitors, or district nurses treating patients in their homes. Nurses may choose to specialize in areas such as accident and emergency, outpatients, operating theatres, and so on. In a hospital, nurses can be appointed to different grades ranging from student nurse to a sister in a ward.

A nurse may often act as the coordinator of care in multidisciplinary teams, so should have good organizational and time management skills, be a good team worker, and have the ability to work on their own initiative. Nurses who have completed a prescribing qualification and a period of learning in practice are able to prescribe medicines.

From 2013 a registered nurse will require 3 years education to degree level and must meet the NMC standards of proficiency for pre-registration nursing education. Students have to be declared as being of good health and good character. Once qualified, the nurse must register with the NMC which maintains a register of nurses who are capable of safe and effective practice.

Occupational therapist

When a person's ability to engage in daily occupations and participate in society is impaired by health or social factors an occupational therapist will perform assessments and work with the person to enable them to maintain, improve, or adapt their skills. Occupational therapists are concerned with the tasks of daily living that cannot be performed due to illness, aging, disability, mental health problems, substance misuse, trauma, poverty, and social exclusion. A pharmacist and an occupational therapist are often part of the same multidisciplinary team.

There are a variety of programmes in the UK which train occupational therapists, most are 3- or 4-year BSc honours degrees, although some universities also offer accelerated 2-year programmes for graduates. Their regulatory body is the HPC.

Optician and optometrist

An optician, also known as a dispensing optician, is a person who is trained to dispense prescriptions for correction of vision. An optician is commonly defined as someone who only makes and dispenses eyeglasses and other eye corrections, and does not perform medical tests. An optician has also been used historically as a term for people skilled in the design or fabrication of all types of optical devices, a field more formally referred to today as optical engineering.

Optometrists (also known as an ophthalmic optician) are the primary health care specialists trained to examine the eyes to detect defects in vision, signs of injury, ocular disease or abnormality, and problems with general health. They might also fit contact lenses and deal with any eye problems that arise.

The training required to become an optometrist is 3 or 4 years' full-time study at university, leading to a degree. This is followed by a further salaried year of clinical experience, after which a qualifying examination is taken before registration with the General Optical Council as an optometrist.

A pharmacist may give advice to an optometrist on medicines management for a patient.

Paramedic

Paramedics are the senior ambulance service health care professionals and are often the first on the scene at an accident or medical emergency. They are normally part of a two-person crew with an ambulance technician to assist them. They assess the patient's condition and then give essential treatment that could potentially save a life. They work closely with doctors and nurses in hospital accident and emergency departments, briefing them as they hand their patient over to their care.

Anyone wishing to work as a paramedic needs to either secure a student paramedic position with an ambulance service trust or attend an approved full-time course in paramedic science at a university. There are a number of higher education institutions that run these and the course is usually 2 years. Their regulatory body is the HPC.

Physiotherapist

Physiotherapists help restore movement and function when someone is affected by injury or illness or by a developmental or other disability. In particular they treat neuromuscular (brain and nervous system), musculoskeletal (soft tissues, joints, and bones), cardiovascular and respiratory systems (heart and lungs and associated physiology). People are usually referred for physiotherapy by doctors or other health and social care professionals. Physiotherapists work in a wide variety of health settings, such as intensive care, mental illness, stroke recovery, occupational health, sports injuries, and care of the elderly.

To become a physiotherapist requires 3 or 4 years of study at a university, which leads to an honours degree in physiotherapy. The training involves periods of theory and clinical placement, including meeting and working with patients. There is also a fast-track course of 27 months at some universities for those with 2 years of work experience in health and social care. The theory part of the course covers anatomy, physiology, physics, and pathology. On placements, students develop communication skills and gain experience of practical treatment. Physiotherapists often treat patients who have pain management issues, and working in a team with a pharmacist can help to provide better care to these patients. Their regulatory body is the HPC.

Podiatrist (chiropodist)

A podiatrist is a specialist devoted to the study, diagnosis, and treatment of disorders of the foot, ankle, and lower leg. The term 'podiatry' came into use in the early twentieth century in the USA. In some areas the specialist term would still be a chiropodist. Podiatrists work in private practice or for the NHS and often visit elderly or housebound patients in their homes. Over 60% of people have foot and lower limb problems during their lifetime and this is when the podiatrist can be a help. They often work in conjunction with GPs and physiotherapists.

To become a podiatrist involves 3 or 4 years' study at a university, with nearly half of the training consisting of practical experience. Their regulatory body is the HPC.

Psychologist

The psychologist's role is to ascertain how the mind works and what motivates people. They specialize in various areas such as mental health work, educational, or occupational psychology. Psychologists are not usually medically qualified and only a small proportion of people studying psychology degrees will go on to work with patients. The majority of graduates entering the NHS will be involved within one of four main specialities: clinical, forensic, health, and counselling.

- A clinical psychologist is a health care professional involved in the treatment of patients with mental health issues. They use their training to understand, relieve, and prevent the psychological distress of patients.

- A forensic psychologist works at the interface of psychology with the legal system and must have a thorough understanding of the law and of courtroom language and etiquette. They are often appointed by the court to assess a defendant's competence to stand trial.

- A health psychologist is a new and evolving role and is mainly concerned with understanding and researching the psychological and cultural factors involved in health and illness.

- A counselling psychologist works therapeutically with clients who present with a variety of mental health problems and difficulties regarding their life.

Training to be a psychologist involves a 3- or 4-year course at university.

Social worker

The International Federation of Social Workers (IFSW) has produced the following definition of social work:

The social work profession promotes social change, problem-solving in human relationships, and the empowerment and liberation of people to enhance well-being. Utilizing theories of human behaviour and social systems, social work intervenes at the points where people interact with their environment. Principles of human rights and social justice are fundamental to social work.

As well as working with a range of different groups, social workers also work in a range of different settings and for a range of different organizations. These include those in the public (local authority/health), voluntary (not for profit), and private (for profit) sectors. Settings include:

- Local authority practice teams
- Hospitals
- Day-care facilities
- Care homes

- Support projects
- Outreach work.

Much social work practice takes place with individuals and families within their own homes; however, work also takes place in settings such as hospitals, prisons, day care, temporary accommodation, supported accommodation, and residential facilities. Social workers and pharmacists may work together in multidisciplinary teams in the care of a patient with mental health or substance misuse issues. Some substance misuse clinics have a pharmacist and pharmacy on site.

There are a number of ways to become a social worker but you need to gain a professional qualification in social work (usually at degree level) either on a full-time or part-time basis. This is offered by universities at an undergraduate and postgraduate level. It is also possible to take a degree course combining social work with mental health or learning disability nursing. To work in the UK a social worker must be registered with the social care council in the relevant home country.

Case study 6.1 invites you to think about the health care professionals who might be involved in caring for an elderly woman with multiple health problems.

SELF CHECK 6.3

Describe the roles of three health and social care professionals who work alongside pharmacists.

107

CASE STUDY 6.1

Mrs Macdonald is 85 years of age and had half of one lung removed 10 years ago. Since that operation she has had mobility problems and has now become virtually housebound. She has a number of comorbidities, including high blood pressure and osteoporosis.

REFLECTION QUESTION

Reading through the list of health care professionals can you identify a number of them who should be involved in Mrs Macdonald's care and why?

Answer
There is no right answer for this question, as most of the health care professions could have an input, but this might vary depending on health board area and on which health care problem was the priority at the time of treatment.

6.3 What is interprofessional education?

Since the 1960s in Britain there have been a number of calls for health and social care professionals to develop better teamworking skills to optimize patient care. This has become increasingly expected in recent years with the recurring shortages of trained health care staff in the NHS. Traditionally, health professionals have not been good at teamworking and collaboration.

Over the intervening decades since the first calls for interprofessional practice a number of short-term initiatives have attempted to address this lack of teamworking. Many of the educational interventions were well developed and organized but had short lifespans mainly owing to changes in the lead staff, lack of funding, or timetabling difficulties. Research has suggested that the way to increase teamworking, and thus improve the quality of patient care, is to develop shared learning programmes at undergraduate level.

Shared learning is the development of collaborative and interactive learning and teaching across a number of health care curricula. It is learning in common with other health and social care students within a multiprofessional framework to develop teamworking and communications skills. Research shows that it is better to develop teamwork and communications skills in health professionals early in their undergraduate education, rather than leave it until they begin their professional careers.

Interprofessional education (IPE) is an interactive development of the more didactic shared learning and has been defined by the Centre for the Advancement of Interprofessional Education as: 'Occasions when two or more professions learn with, from and about each other to improve collaboration and the quality of care.'

 See Chapter 2 for more information on the organization of health care in the UK.

SELF CHECK 6.4

Explain what is meant by the term 'interprofessional education'.

Why interprofessional education?

In the current health care system, patients are increasingly cared for by multidisciplinary teams involving a wide range of health care and other professionals. It is therefore vital that effective teamworking, collaboration, and communication exist across professional boundaries, ensuring high-quality care that benefits patients. IPE between different professions is a means of achieving such teamworking.

It has been shown that effective teamwork can improve the quality of patient care. However, until recent years there has been little focus on this area in pre-registration health and social care curricula. As a result of this many students have entered the workforce poorly prepared for the challenges associated with working in multidisciplinary teams. It is therefore logical to suggest that if people are expected to work in teams they should be educated in teams. IPE between health care professions has been shown to develop more positive attitudes, to demonstrate the importance of multiprofessional teamwork and communication, and to increase knowledge and understanding of other health care professions. There is also widespread acceptance that undergraduate interprofessional learning is perceived as beneficial by the NHS and the students involved—removing stereotypes and enhancing communication and teamwork skills between different health professions. Research has suggested that the way forward to improve teamworking, and thus improve the quality of patient care, is to develop IPE programmes as early as possible at an undergraduate level.

Problem-based learning

Teaching in lecture format to different multiprofessional groups has never been perceived as the best way forward for interprofessional learning to impact on working practice, mainly because the students do not get a chance to interact or develop teamworking skills. Normally, interprofessional learning uses some variation of **problem-based learning**. This is an instructional method that challenges students to 'learn to learn' by working cooperatively in small groups to seek solutions to problems. It is a very useful technique within a number of health and social care courses. Problem-based learning encourages discussion and decision-making, often in team settings. This helps students to develop collaboration and negotiation skills from their own experience of teamworking in their undergraduate courses. This is based loosely on the theories of educationalist David Kolb. It allows the development of the necessary skills for team-based decision-making and is therefore a very useful type of learning to develop interprofessional practice. A number of advocates of IPE and interprofessional practice have used problem-based learning and experiential learning to develop their interprofessional learning provision.

SELF CHECK 6.5

Describe problem-based learning.

6.4 UK initiatives in interprofessional education

In the last 10 years there have been a number of initiatives throughout the UK that have focused on the development of interprofessional education at an undergraduate level. These have been different in each of the four countries of the UK. Since political devolution in the 1990s, the health and education systems in each of the countries have developed in a variety of ways and the development of IPE has differed in each area. However, the need for IPE is the same in all of them.

After the Wanless Report in 2002 concluded that health care was going to become increasingly costly for the UK as a whole, each of the four countries became interested in the development of self-care programmes for patients and the coproduction of services and care. Other themes that emerged were integrated service delivery across health and social care and making the most of the skills of the whole clinical team. IPE was in position to become one of the foremost educational movements of the twenty-first century to promote better (and therefore hopefully more financially efficient) patient care.

One issue has been the sustainability of IPE initiatives once the central funding has disappeared, leaving universities to take financial as well as organizational control. 'Champions for IPE' have been appointed in many universities and it is their role to take the now unfunded projects forward and to make them sustainable for the future.

England

Four large IPE projects lasting for 3 years or more were funded by the government in England in 2002.

The first of these projects was developed by Newcastle, Northumbria, and Teesside Universities with the workforce development confederations for the North of England and for County Durham and Tees Valley. This project was to develop and implement practice-based interprofessional learning. The professions involved were medicine, nursing, speech and language therapy, occupational therapy, physiotherapy, and social work. They found a number of problems and over the period of the project the type of practice placements changed. There were no pharmacists involved in this project. The project developed and tested three models of IPE in practice for small numbers of students from seven professions at Newcastle, Northumbria, and Teesside Universities. All three models focused on providing students with an experience of working in teams which shadowed actual practice. Teams were identified in which practice teachers from different professions were located and which also included one or more placement students. Appropriate clients were selected by the staff and students for an interprofessional case study. It was felt that the three models might be appropriate to encourage flexibility in an NHS already beset by resource constraints.

109

The second project was in the south-east of London and involved King's College London, London South Bank University, and Greenwich University with South East London Workforce Development Confederation. This project was again involved in trying to develop IPE in a practice setting. It found that the large numbers of students (over 7000 at any one time), the professional body requirement for diverse placements, and the length of placements caused a number of difficulties. The model devised enabled groups of students from different professions to follow a patient's journey through his or her eyes. The programme was piloted in one hospital before being extended to others and then to primary care. Half the target number of students was reached within the 2-year life of the programme. As a result, IPE became more serendipitous than planned, except for medical and nursing students.

The third project, developed by Sheffield and Sheffield Hallam Universities with the South Yorkshire Workforce Development Confederation, represented another practice-based IPE initiative between the two universities. It included dentistry, medicine, nursing, social work, occupational therapy, physiotherapy, and paramedics. Five 'beacon' sites were selected which would offer students on placement the experience of user-centred collaborative working attuned to the NHS's modernization agenda. A significant advance was the development of an 'interprofessional capability framework', which others have adopted at home and abroad to use in the development of IPE.

The last project, in Southampton and Portsmouth Universities with the Hampshire and Isle of Wight Workforce Development Confederation, was the largest and best-funded. The curriculum changes involved in the New Generation Project were launched in 2003 and remain in place. The project comprises 'common learning' within three undergraduate interprofessional learning units, which are mandatory, assessed, and embedded within all pre-qualifying health and social care programmes, with 1500 students per intake. The professions involved are audiology, diagnostic radiography, medicine, midwifery, nursing, occupational therapy, pharmacy, physiotherapy, social work, and therapeutic radiography.

Each of these four projects followed very different models of IPE and each conducted its own evaluation in accordance with its agreement with the Department of Health. There have been a number of journal and Internet articles published as a result of these projects.

Scotland

Scotland historically has different education and health systems and, although following a similar timeframe, the initiatives have been more piecemeal than in England. In his foreword to a 2002 publication from the Scottish Executive, *The Right Medicine: A Strategy for Pharmaceutical Care in Scotland*, the Chief Pharmaceutical Officer for Scotland stated: 'Whole system working and improving the patient's experience within and across clinical and organizational boundaries sets a challenge to health care professionals.' Only one project has been funded in Scotland and that was the IPE initiative in Aberdeen between Robert Gordon University and the University of Aberdeen. The focus has been on the development of a flexible IPE programme with large- and small-scale interactions as well as short placement experiences, online buddy groups, and case-based scenarios. Ten professions are involved: medicine, pharmacy, diagnostic radiography, physiotherapy, nursing, midwifery, occupational therapy, nutrition, dietetics, and social work. There are also plans to include police cadets and student teachers.

There were a number of other smaller initiatives in Edinburgh, Dundee, and Glasgow but without the numbers or the sustainability involved in the Aberdeen project.

Wales and Northern Ireland

In Wales there have been 13 small localized IPE events but around half of these are at postgraduate level. In Northern Ireland most IPE is at postgraduate level.

Outside the UK

IPE is not limited to the UK; there are a number of initiatives throughout the English-speaking world, notably Australasia, North America, and the Nordic countries, generating opportunities to share experience and to learn from each other.

6.5 Is interprofessional education effective?

Over the last 10 years the evidence for IPE and its effectiveness has grown exponentially. A systematic review published in 2005 concluded that IPE did have the capacity 'to help improve collaborative practice and … to improve the quality of care'. Students enjoy their IPE experiences at university and often cite these as some of the most enjoyable and beneficial interactions they have with other students. Comments such as: 'shows strengths and weaknesses of both professions' and 'pooled knowledge of both groups combined is infinitely better than the individual knowledge of each group, which ultimately leads to better patient care' are often quoted at the end of IPE sessions.

Within universities interprofessionalism can work well. However, the workplace can be a different prospect for many students and many of the professionals that the students meet will have come from a very different way of working and practice. Students need to appreciate that while it is relatively easy to create an interprofessional working space in a controlled environment, this can be more problematic once out in the 'real world' of work. For IPE to be effective a workforce needs to be committed to working together for the benefit not only of itself but ultimately for the patient. While there may not yet be the longitudinal studies that prove that IPE is effective, high-profile inquiries after tragic deaths nearly always recommend that the best way to achieve better patient care is effective teamworking.

As interprofessional education has become more important during the last decade so has the fear that this could be a way for the government and the NHS to develop a new role—that of the generic health and social care worker who would be able to take on the responsibilities of a number of professions, thus negating the need for the trained specialist. This has not been the case, yet the fear of this happening has coloured some of the approaches to interprofessional working over the last few years.

The next 10 years will show whether IPE will be able to continue in the climate of reduced funding, and whether the evidence base can be increased to provide stronger foundations to help sustain the higher education initiatives. Perhaps one of the main concerns with IPE is the question of whether it is an effective response to improve patient care in the future.

6.6 What is interprofessional working?

Once a student leaves the confines of the university at the end of their degree, or when they are out on placement, the reality of the workplace is often that postgraduate teams do not work as well as all would hope. Entrenched professional stereotypes and prejudices become more apparent and can cause dysfunctional teams and poor teamworking. Interprofessional working is when all team members work with each other—when there is adequate and appropriate communication and respect for the other professions.

What specialist skills do teams need to work interprofessionally? The foundation is always communication, which involves all of the team in processing complex information in a way that acquires meaning for them as a professional but also as a member of the inter-agency team. Hopefully the development and proliferation of interprofessional education will allow the development of a mindset or a framework that helps to organize the meaning of every interprofessional encounter.

The 'five Cs'

The 'five Cs' that are fundamental to the creation of a successful team are:

- *Communication*: every member of the team has to communicate not only with their peers but also

111

with the levels above and below to let all know what is happening and what is being achieved within the team. All communication needs to be appropriate for the situation.

- *Consistency*: there needs to be a consistency of approach by all the team members and a consistency as to how they are treated and how they treat others in that role.

- *Commitment*: all team members must have a commitment to the improvement of patient care as well as an improvement of interprofessional working.

- *Clarity*: there needs to be clarity of the professional role and also of the role that the professional plays in the team. This needs to be clearly demonstrated throughout all the team discussions and interactions. Blurred boundaries of professional responsibility do not help in the creation of clarity.

- *Clear direction*: the team members need to know what their goals are and how these can be achieved by all working together.

An awareness of the five Cs as well as the commitment to using them as you progress through your course will allow you to develop as an effective health care practitioner.

Terminology

A multidisciplinary team will include health and social care professionals from a number of specialities brought together to provide seamless care for an individual. The terminology that is used by each member of that team can differ; for example, an individual might be referred to as a 'patient', 'service user', 'client', or even a 'customer'. It is important that this does not cause problems within teams. When you have several professions working together using one set of case notes they still might not all understand all of the information. Each professional group has its own set of acronyms; for example, 'CPR' can be 'cardiopulmonary resuscitation' to one set of health care professionals but 'child protection register' to others, and 'UTI' might refer to a 'urinary tract infection' or an 'unexplained traumatic injury'. Therefore, one of the first rules of multidisciplinary teams is to make sure that

they all use the same shorthand terms or acronyms; otherwise there is chance of confusion occurring inadvertently.

Other terms for multidisciplinary teams include partnership working, multiagency working, interprofessional collaboration, inter-agency coordination, integrated teams, interdisciplinary teams, or collaborative relationships.

KEY POINT

One of the first ground rules for any multidisciplinary team working together is to make sure that they use the same shorthand terms for treatment and illnesses.

Barriers to good teamwork

While there are a number of imperatives that have aided the development of interprofessional working there are also a number of barriers that need to be addressed. These can be divided into three main groups: personal, professional, and political.

- Personal barriers that can stop teams working well together can be caused by something as fundamental as personality clashes or staff with different values and attitudes.

- Professional barriers can be different understandings of terminology, of client needs, or of organizational structures.

- Political barriers are those of organizational priorities, policies, and procedures, and of leadership.

Once these barriers are understood and identified then teams can begin to work together to resolve the issues.

It is often asked how the practice of interprofessional working can develop in the future. Evidence would suggest that the instillation of interprofessional values from the early stages of university education, reinforced by interprofessional practice placements, will be the way to create a workforce that respects and values other health and social care professionals. These collaborative professionals will be the building blocks for an interprofessional workforce of the future.

6.7 Communication with patients: the development of the art of consultation

The consultation has always been the basic tool of doctors in general practice. It has evolved over the years, with many factors contributing to changes in consultation styles, content, and length. In the early days of the NHS patients did not usually have booked appointment times and queued to see the doctor; because of staff shortages appointments were very short. The 1960s and 1970s saw the advent of allocated appointment times, with each patient allocated 5 min. Today, the *Quality and Outcomes Framework* demands consultations at 10-minute intervals. In one study in the UK, average consultation lengths were 8 min. Patients with psychosocial problems were given 1 minute longer on average and this was sufficient to improve quality of care. Patients continue to express dissatisfaction with the time spent with their GP.

New models of care have developed in the last decade with the advent of non-medical prescribers: pharmacists and nurses able to diagnose conditions and prescribe medicines. These patient consultations are often for 20–30 min and patient satisfaction has increased because they feel they are given more time to discuss their condition/s and understand their illness and their medication. Increasing the length of consultations is not the only important consideration; the development of better consultation skills is also important to all health and social care professionals who are involved in discussing treatment or care with patients.

Consultation skills

Consultations have been studied and analysed by a variety of people over the years, usually highlighting similar conclusions. The main literature base for any discussion of consultation skills started in the late 1950s with the work of Michael and Enid Balint, two psychoanalysts working in London.

 See the 'Further reading' section for notable contributions to the literature on understanding and analysing the consultation.

The consultation is divided into the following sections, which provide structure and allow signposting of the topics:

- Initiating the session (rapport, reasons for consulting, establishing shared agenda).
- Gathering information (patient's story, open and closed questions, identifying verbal and non-verbal cues).
- Building the relationship (developing rapport, recording notes, accepting patient's views/feelings and demonstrating empathy and support).
- Explanation and planning (giving digestible information and explanations).
- Closing the session (summarizing and clarifying the agreed plan).

An open question is one where the interviewer does not give any indication of the type of response required and allows the patient to use their own words and experience to structure the response. For example, 'tell me how your pain medication has affected your quality of life.' A closed question would be where you want a short, usually factual, response; for example, 'what pain medication do you take?' There is a place for both in any consultation but the closed questions often set the framework whereas the open questions will explore deeper and richer issues.

Using body-language techniques such as verbal and non-verbal cues are also important in discerning responses to questions. When patients perhaps seem unhappy or nervous about their answers this might indicate that they are not giving all the relevant information and it would be up to the interviewer to probe deeper. One of the best ways to develop rapport with patients is to address them as an individual, introduce yourself, and explain why you are speaking to them. Once the scene setting has happened it is up to the health care professional as interviewer to ask appropriate questions, listen to the response, and make sure that the next question flows logically from the patient's response. Smiling and having eye contact as well as indicating that you are listening are all helpful in creating rapport with the patient.

A number of health and social care professionals use the Calgary–Cambridge model (Box 6.2, Case Studies 6.2 and 6.3), especially those such as non-medical prescribers where medical mentors are involved in the training and it is appropriate to be using similar consultation models.

The models of consultation skills listed in the 'Further reading' section give a useful guide to developing an interest in individual patient concerns and encouraging patients to become more involved in the decision-making, thus hopefully increasing their adherence with particular therapies or drug regimens. This does not mean that practitioners give away all responsibility but rather the consultation becomes a shared process, with both parties involved, thus increasing satisfaction with the consultation and the adherence of the patient to the treatment.

 See Chapter 5 for more information on prescribing and dispensing.

BOX 6.2

The Calgary–Cambridge model

The Calgary–Cambridge method of analysing consultations is used by a large number of medical, nursing, and pharmacy schools in the UK to teach communication skills. This method is an evidence-based approach to integrating the 'tasks' of the consultation and improving skills for effective communication. Methods used include role play with fellow students, interactions with volunteer patients, and critiquing video recordings of your own or others' interactions.

The model, developed by Kurtz and Silverman in 1996, provides an easy-to-use structure which includes elements that have their origins in the traditional holistic approach of nurses. The focus is on building a relationship with the patient as part of the consultation progresses. In this model the consultation is divided into six stages, which can be summarized as follows:

1. Preparing the environment—establishing initial rapport with the patient and identifying the reason(s) for the consultation.

2. Exploring the problem by gathering information from the practitioner and the patient perspective to set it in context.

3. Building the relationship and establishing the patient involvement.

4. Providing structure and signposting to the interview.

5. Explaining the process and achieving a shared understanding.

6. Closing the interview and developing a forward plan.

CASE STUDY 6.2

As a pharmacist you run a hypertension clinic within a GP surgery and Mr Rashid, aged 41, has been referred to the clinic by his GP.

REFLECTION QUESTION

What steps would you use to conduct this initial interview?

Answer

You should use the model set by the Calgary–Cambridge method as described in Box 6.2, making sure that you are listening to Mr Rashid's responses.

As a pharmacist you run a hypertension clinic within a GP surgery and Mr Rashid, aged 41, has been referred to the clinic by his GP. On his second visit to the clinic 6 months later you discover that he has not been taking the medication as prescribed.

> **REFLECTION QUESTION**
>
> If Mr Rashid was not taking his medication as prescribed what could you do about this?

Answer

You have to ask Mr Rashid why this is the case without sounding as if you are judging him adversely. Once you have discerned the issues—whether it be he did not understand how to take the medicine, or he felt unwell after taking it, or someone had told him that he did not need it—you then have to advise him of the need to take his medicine, how to take it, and why it is important. Help him in more practical ways if you can, for example by helping him set an alarm on his phone to remind him to take the medicine.

These consultation structures, developed since the 1950s, have aimed to achieve a better partnership between health professional and patient, which should in the long run result in better patient care and better outcomes. The core tasks in any consultation have been defined as follows:

- Identification of the patient's main problem.
- Development of a holistic assessment which encompasses the physical, emotional, and social impact.

KEY POINT

A consultation should develop a **holistic** assessment of the patient and their main problem. This should encompass not only the physical impact but also the emotional and social.

SELF CHECK 6.6

List the six stages within the Calgary–Cambridge method.

115

6.8 Concordance and adherence from the patient perspective

Persuading patients to take their prescribed medicines has long been regarded as problematic. However, non-compliance often has serious and wide-reaching outcomes, not only for the patient and their treatment but also for the inappropriate use of medications, which can result in drug wastage. **Concordance** is a way of looking at the processes within the consultation, allowing the patient's agenda to be taken into account when reaching a management decision. This approach to the prescribing and taking of medicines was developed in the early 2000s. It is an agreement reached after negotiation between a patient and a health care professional that respects the beliefs and wishes of the patient in determining whether, when, and how medicines are to be taken and the reasons for this type of treatment. This allows the patient to be primarily included in the decision-making process about taking the recommended medications.

 See Chapter 5 for more information on prescribing and dispensing and Chapter 7 for information on how the behavioural and social sciences relate to the practice of pharmacy.

CHAPTER SUMMARY

➤ There have been a number of high-profile cases with tragic consequences where failure in communication between different professions has been implicated.

➤ The health care team is composed of many different professions that can interact with pharmacists.

➤ Interprofessional education is where two or more professions learn with and about each other and there have

been a number of pilot schemes throughout the UK. Many of these have involved problem-based learning.

➤ Effective teamwork relies on the five Cs—good communication, consistency, commitment, clarity, and clear direction.

➤ Developing effective communication skills is a key part of the concordance approach.

FURTHER READING

Health and Care Professions Council. <http://www.hpc-uk.org>.

> The HPC is the regulatory body for many of the professions discussed in this chapter.

Coster, S., D'Avray, L., Dawson, P., et al. Barr H. (Ed.) *Piloting Interprofessional Education: Four English Case Studies.* Occasional Paper 8. Higher Education Academy, 2007. <http://eprints.soton.ac.uk/49350/>.

> In 2007 a review of the UK IPE pilots was written by Hugh Barr for the Higher Education Academy and further details of each pilot can be found at this website.

Centre for the Advancement of Interprofessional Education (CAIPE) 2002. http://www.caipe.org.uk/ [Accessed 27 November 2011].

> The Centre for the Advancement of Interprofessional Education provides a number of articles and reports focusing on interprofessional education which can be downloaded.

Lord Laming. *The Victoria Climbié Inquiry: Report of an Inquiry by Lord Laming.* HMSO, 2003.

> The official report of the inquiry into the death of Victoria Climbié.

O'Brien S. *The Caleb Ness Inquiry: Report of an Inquiry by Susan O'Brien, QC.* Edinburgh: HMSO, 2003.

> The official report of the inquiry into the death of Caleb Ness.

Kennedy, I. *Final Report: Bristol Royal Infirmary Inquiry.* HMSO, 2001.

> The official report of the inquiry into children's heart surgery at Bristol Royal Infirmary.

Balint, M. *The Doctor, The Patient and His Illness.* Churchill Livingstone, 1957.

> Balint describes how attentive listening helped make patients feel better. Balint describes listening as a skill and holds that 'asking questions only gets you answers'.

Byrne, P. and Long, B. *Doctors Talking to Patients.* RCGP, 1976.

> The authors recognize that doctors have tended to use a narrow repertoire of consultation skills and that those who ask more open questions tend to see their patients less frequently.

Pendleton, D., Schofield, T., Tate, P., and Havelock, P. *The New Consultation: Developing Doctor–Patient Communication.* OUP, 2003.

> Pendleton, a social psychologist who wrote his PhD thesis on analysis of the consultation, has had a great influence on subsequent work and thinking. His great addition to the consultation skill was to develop the use of video and the rules and etiquette of recording consultations.

Tate, P. *The Doctor's Communication Handbook.* 5th edn. Radcliffe, 2007.

> Tate developed some of his themes from work with David Pendleton. He was responsible for the introduction of a video module to MRCGP (Membership of the Royal College of General Practitioners) examinations in 1996 and he emphasizes the importance of the patient's agenda, particularly their ideas, concerns, and expectations.

Royal College of General Practitioners. *The Future General Practitioner.* RCGP, 1972.

> This book marked the start of work by many within the RCGP that helped define general practice and included consideration of the physical, psychological, and social condition of the patient.

Kurtz, S.M. and Silverman, J.D. The Calgary–Cambridge Referenced Observation Guides: An aid to defining the curriculum and organizing the teaching in communication training programmes. *Medical Education* 1996; 30: 83–9.

> The Calgary–Cambridge method is an evidence-based approach to integration of the 'tasks' of the consultation and improving skills for effective communication. It is now used by a large number of medical, nursing, and pharmacy schools in the UK.

7 Behavioural and social sciences

JANE SUTTON

As earlier chapters in this book have described, pharmacists contribute to the health care of patients through their expertise as medicines specialists. They generally do this as part of a multidisciplinary team that can include doctors, nurses, paramedics, physiotherapists, radiographers, dieticians, occupational therapists, and psychologists. There are a number of different types of psychologist, some of whom work directly with patients to help resolve problems (clinical psychologists). Others, such as health psychologists, not only work directly with patients but also study factors which affect health, such as models of disease causation and people's beliefs about illness and health. The science of psychology is known as a behavioural science, and alongside the social sciences can contribute to our understanding of factors that affect health and how we might use this understanding to help people to attain and maintain an optimum individual level of health. This chapter seeks to provide an introduction to what behavioural and social scientists do, and considers how specialist knowledge of health psychology issues can help pharmacists to better understand health behaviours.

We have already touched on a couple of areas associated with behavioural and social sciences. In Chapter 5 we talked about the terms 'adherence', 'compliance', and 'concordance'. These all relate to whether or not people take medicines that have been prescribed for them. If people are not taking their medicines then this may mean that their condition could deteriorate. If, as pharmacists, we can understand why people are not taking their medicine we can try to find ways to help them understand why the taking of their medicine is beneficial.

Learning objectives

Having read this chapter you are expected to be able to:

➤ Describe the behavioural and social sciences.

➤ Describe some of the definitions of health.

➤ Understand the role of health psychology.

➤ Understand how models of health behaviour can contribute to health care.

➤ List ways that health and health inequalities might be measured.

➤ Relate theories of health behaviour to pharmacy practice.

➤ Discuss gender and cultural differences in health.

➤ Describe illness behaviour and the rights and obligations of patients and health care professionals.

➤ Explore lay views of health, illness, disease, and medicines.

➤ Understand how research methods in social sciences can contribute to pharmacy practice research.

7.1 What are the behavioural and social sciences?

The terms 'behavioural science' and 'social science' are often confused with each other. They are related because they are both concerned with the study of human behaviour. However, they differ in that they 'work' at different levels of analysis of various dimensions of behaviour.

- *Behavioural science*: This is concerned with the activities and interactions among human beings in a social system. This includes the discipline of psychology.
- *Social science*: This provides a framework for studying the processes that go on in a social system and how these affect the broader organization of society as a whole. Social science includes sociology, economics, and anthropology.

In this chapter we are going to talk mostly about behavioural science and in particular a branch of psychology called health psychology. This is because it is the behavioural science that has most relevance to pharmacy practice in helping us to make sense of what people do and why. First, however, let's think about health itself as a concept.

 You might want to go back to Chapter 4 at this point and revise how health is commonly defined before we look at some ways of conceptualizing health in Section 7.2.

7.2 Definitions of health and illness

As human beings we are all different. Not only do we physically come in different shapes and sizes, we think and feel about things differently. These differences are caused by many factors: our varied experiences, ideas we have picked up from family and friends, and so on. We all have a unique definition of what 'being healthy' or 'being ill' means to us and by considering these definitions, we can begin to think about and understand what they might mean to others (see Case Study 7.1).

We tend almost to stereotype people when we are describing whether they are healthy or not, and often get a mental picture of a 'type' of person; for example, thin, fat, muscular, rosy-cheeked. Table 7.1 shows

CASE STUDY 7.1

Naina Patel is 51 years of age and was diagnosed with type 2 diabetes mellitus when she was aged 45. Type 2 diabetes is a condition whereby the body develops resistance to insulin, which disturbs its ability to process sugar. Diet, lifestyle, and medication can help to control the condition.

REFLECTION QUESTION

Would you classify Mrs Patel as 'ill' or 'healthy'?

Answer

There is no right or wrong answer because all patients with acute or chronic illnesses still have some degree of health in terms of physical, mental, spiritual, and social well-being. However, the way you perceive the health of others may affect the way you approach patients or members of the public when you practice as a pharmacist. Research by Ogden et al. (2001) suggests that doctors and patients do not always have the same understanding of health and that this can have implications for primary care consultations. Similarly, pharmacists carry out consultations, each time they interact with a patient or member of the public, so a shared understanding of health can be useful in establishing a good therapeutic relationship. As a pharmacist it is your role in advising patients to help them improve their health and help them to live within the bounds of their condition.

TABLE 7.1 Popular definitions of health

Definition	Description
Health as not ill	Absence of physical symptoms
Health despite disease	Has an illness or condition which is under control
Health as reserve	Comes from a 'strong' family; recovered quickly from an operation
Health as behaviour	Usually applied to others; for example, that person is healthy because they exercise regularly
Health as physical fitness	Male health concept more tied to feeling 'fit'
Health as vitality	More a female health concept
Health as psychosocial well-being	Free from mental health problems and interacts well with others
Health as social relationships	Spends time with friends, joins in with social activities
Health as function	Physical health, the body is in 'working order'

some popular definitions of health, with definitions that might help your understanding of it.

Factors affecting health

There are a number of factors that contribute to our health and well-being. Some of these are beyond our control (for example, genetic factors) but others are related to our lifestyle or behaviour and can be adapted or changed under some circumstances.

- *Genetic*: Some people are born with a tendency to develop a particular condition. Some conditions and diseases 'run in families' and so members of these families may be at a higher level of physiological risk than other members of the population; for example, ovarian cancer.

- *Environmental*: People who live in poverty or in polluted environments tend to be more at risk of developing health problems. For example, people who live in overcrowded, poorly maintained housing may be more at risk of contracting tuberculosis.

- *Lifestyle*: The way we live our lives and our behaviour can also affect our health. Decreased use of tobacco, regular exercise, and a well-balanced diet can help us to maintain good health. On the other hand, being overweight and engaging in unsafe sexual activity can have the opposite effect.

- *Psychosocial*: Research has shown (Wade and Kendler, 2000) that poor social support and poor coping skills can affect the way we cope with illness, and in some people can lead to isolation and a decrease in mental health.

Pharmacists are in a prime position to be able to help people improve or maintain their health; those who work in community pharmacies are often the first health care professional a person will go to if they have a health concern. It is the pharmacist's role to provide health counselling and other services (as well as advice on medications), so it is important that you learn how people's behaviour can affect health and what you can do to help. You may even go on to train as a pharmacist independent prescriber, in which case you will need to understand much more about the people you are caring for.

Psychological theory, as it relates to health, can contribute to our understanding of why people do things that have the potential to make them ill even when they know it is bad for them. This is an area of applied psychology called health psychology, which we will look at in Section 7.3.

7.3 What is health psychology?

Marks et al. (2000) describe health psychology as: 'an interdisciplinary field concerned with the application of psychological knowledge and techniques to health, illness and health care'.

Health psychology is concerned with human behaviour and its effect on health. Its primary aim is to help answer some of the following questions:

- What causes illness?
- Who is responsible for illness?
- How should illness be treated?
- Who is responsible for treatment?
- What is the relationship between health and illness?
- What is the role of psychology in health and illness?

KEY POINT

A knowledge of health psychology can help us to understand, explain, develop, and test theories. An understanding of theories about health can enable us to evaluate the role of behaviours and to predict unhealthy behaviours.

From a treatment point of view, developing an understanding of the role of psychology in the experience of illness, and evaluating that role, can contribute to the way we design interventions to encourage people to change their behaviours in order to prevent ill health and promote good health. As a pharmacist it is important that you understand some of these theories too. They will help you to understand why some interventions work for some people but not for all. The reason for this is simple—we are all individuals with our own reasons for doing the things we do, and they make perfect sense to us!

Beliefs about illness and health

Why do people do things they know are bad for them and how can we as health care professionals make sense of that behaviour? Before we go any further have a look at Case Study 7.2.

KEY POINT

We must accept that patients and members of the public have beliefs about all sorts of things to do with their health and just because we do not understand them it does not mean that they are not important and legitimate to each individual.

 Chapter 5 (section 5.10, 'Giving the medicine to the patient') considers how we can communicate with patients to ensure that we understand them and they understand us.

CASE STUDY 7.2

Mahendra Patel was diagnosed with high blood pressure last year but doesn't take her medication unless her daughter-in-law Naina is around to remind her. When Naina sat her down and asked her why she often missed taking her medication Mrs Patel revealed that she was actually frightened of 'those nasty red pills'.

REFLECTION QUESTION

If you were Mrs Patel's pharmacist what might your reaction be? What information would be important to get from Mrs Patel?

Answer

All of us who work in the health care professions are guilty of assuming that we are right and that we know best when it comes to appropriate treatment. We might even think that Mrs Patel's beliefs about red tablets are ridiculous. However, until we understand why Mrs Patel is frightened of taking the tablets we cannot begin to provide the tailored information she needs, which will hopefully lead to her taking the blood pressure medication without Naina having to prompt her. A knowledge of health psychology and how people develop beliefs about illness and health can therefore help us to understand and to take action to improve things like Mrs Patel's adherence to her medication. She might even live longer if you, as a pharmacist, can help bring her blood pressure down.

7.4 Models of health behaviour and their contribution to health care

Models of health behaviour help us to understand why we do things that affect our health. For the purpose of this chapter we will focus on five definitions of health behaviour.

The first three were defined by Kasl and Cobb in 1966:

- A health behaviour is a behaviour aimed at preventing disease (for example, taking regular exercise).

- An illness behaviour is a behaviour aimed at seeking a remedy (for example, going to see a health care professional such as a doctor or pharmacist).

- A sick role behaviour is any activity aimed at getting well (for example, taking medicines as prescribed).

Later on, in 1984, Matarazzo suggested two further health behaviours:

- Behavioural pathogens are health-impairing habits (for example, smoking or drinking too much alcohol).

- Behavioural immunogens are health-protective behaviours (for example, having regular health checks).

There are many more ways that health-related behaviours have been defined and you can find more information on this if you go to the resources suggested in the 'Further reading' section.

The health models are also known as **cognition** models of health behaviour because their basic assumption is that the way we think about things to do

with our health affects our behaviour. There is a core assumption in the models that our beliefs about health affect our behaviour over time. It may also be possible that if we do something often enough and long enough it can also affect our beliefs (Case Study 7.3).

> ### KEY POINT
>
> Human behaviour happens as a result of our experiences and attitudes that develop over time. As such we may not be aware that the beliefs and attitudes we hold exist and are affecting our behaviour.

In the rest of this section we will look at some of the main models of health behaviour.

The health belief model

The health belief model (HBM) may be described as the process of 'weighing up' the pros and cons of carrying out an action that will have an impact on health. There are a number of components to the HBM, including **demographics** (see Figure 7.1). The other components are explained in Table 7.2 and are applied to a person considering giving up smoking.

Sometimes we deliberate things like this quite consciously and for a long time. At other times, however, things can happen to us or other people that have an immediate effect on us and these are called cues to action. They can lead us to change our behaviour without going through the deliberation process. You

CASE STUDY 7.3

Raj Patel is a fitness fanatic—he believes that to be 'healthy' he has got to go to the gym three to four times a week. He is now 28 years of age and has been going to the gym regularly since he was 16 and has a great physique. It is possible that the fact that he keeps his body in good shape and feels good about it perpetuates his belief that exercise is 'good for you'.

REFLECTION QUESTION

Can you think of something you do because of a firmly held belief? Do you think that as a result of that behaviour your beliefs are strengthened or changed?

FIGURE 7.1 The health belief model
Source: Rosenstock et al., 1994

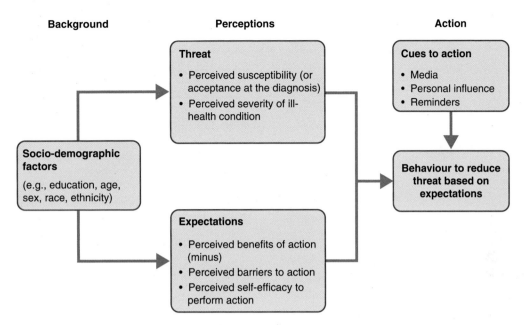

will see from the diagram that there is an arrow going straight from 'cues to action' to 'health behaviour'.

According to the model there are two types of cues to action:

- *Internal cues*: such as experiencing breathlessness when doing something that would not normally cause such symptoms.

- *External cues*: such as being given a leaflet about stopping smoking, which has the effect of convincing you to give up smoking immediately (see Case Study 7.4).

On the whole the HBM is a useful framework for investigating health behaviours. It has been used successfully to explore the prediction of whether or not women do breast self-examination to detect changes that might indicate breast cancer. Norman and Brain (2005) used a questionnaire that was based on the HBM and measured the components discussed. They found that there was an association between the frequency of breast self-examination and perceived emotional barriers, which are included in the perceived barriers that might prevent people from making changes to their health-related behaviour.

TABLE 7.2 Components of the health belief model

Component	Definition	Application to smoker
Perceived susceptibility	How susceptible to the disease a person thinks they are	The smoker sees a 'stop smoking' advert on the television. They understand that because they smoke their chances of getting lung cancer are higher than if they were a non-smoker
Perceived severity	A person's belief about the seriousness of the health effects of smoking	The smoker feels that lung cancer is a serious illness
Perceived benefits	The things that a person sees as incentives to giving up smoking	The smoker knows that quitting smoking will save money
Perceived barriers	The things that a person might perceive as stopping them from giving up	The smoker's friends also smoke, so they worry that peer-group pressure might prevent them from succeeding
Health motivation	What drives a person to a change of behaviour	The smoker is motivated to give up smoking as they recognize the overwhelming benefits it would make to their long-term health

Sarah, aged 19, is back from university for the weekend. Her mother, Naina, is doing some washing for her and finds a packet of cigarettes in her pocket. Naina confronts Sarah, who admits that she has one 'now and again'. She understands that it is bad for her health but doesn't like to feel left out from her friends, some of whom are smokers.

REFLECTION QUESTIONS

1. Thinking about the HBM, if Sarah came into your pharmacy and told you this what do you think you might say?

2. There have been some criticisms of the HBM. Look at the model and see if you can work out what these might be.

Answers

1 You could ask Sarah about her smoking and find out a bit more about when she started to smoke; she might reveal how much she is actually smoking. You could also talk to her about her friends who smoke and explore the ideas that she might not feel accepted by her peers if she does not smoke. You could also talk to her about the non-health benefits of not smoking; for example having more money.

2

- The model assumes that all health behaviours are conscious, but some are not. Things we do every day become automatic; for example, tooth brushing.
- The model places emphasis on the individual but we live in a social world and other people can affect the way we behave. The model does not include social factors.
- The model does not include emotional factors; for example, fear and denial.

But:

- HBM is a useful framework for investigating health behaviours.
- It can be modified to include other components; for example, health motivation and perceived control (self-efficacy) have been added to the model.

The theory of planned behaviour

As with the HBM, the theory of planned behaviour (TPB) attempts to link our beliefs or attitudes with our behaviour.

The TPB says that there are three factors—attitude, subjective norm, and perceived behavioural control—that predict our intention to behave in a certain way, and that those intentions predict actual behaviours. Of course we all know that that may not be the case; we only have to think about all those broken New Year's resolutions that seemed such a good idea at midnight on 31 December!

Using Case Study 7.4 we can see how this might work in practice. Sarah is invited to go on holiday but has to pay for it herself.

- *Attitude*: Sarah's attitude may be that giving up smoking will mean she has more money and she values that money (and the holiday) more than she does the smoking.

- *Subjective norm*: An aspect of the TPB model is that individuals must believe that their actions are valued by others. So perhaps Sarah really cares about what her parents think, and so giving up smoking would really please her mum.

- *Perceived behavioural control*: The final component of the model is that for people to act on their beliefs the actual action must be possible because they have access to the resources that might help. So if Sarah has been given a leaflet about smoking cessation by her pharmacist she will know that she can get help with her craving for nicotine.

In the same way that the HBM says that cues to action can have a direct effect on behaviour the TPB says that perceived behavioural control can have a direct effect too. That is, the action can take place without it being mediated by the intention.

The TPB has been widely tested using health research and successfully applied to real-life practice (we will look at the role of research at the end of this chapter). The model builds in those things that happen in our minds that influence behaviour; for example, beliefs. The model also acknowledges that the role of social pressure is important and that our perceived behavioural control includes the role of past behaviour. The TPB has also been used to explore why young people do/do not engage in safe sex.

SELF CHECK 7.1

As you might expect, there have been criticisms of this model too. Think about what these might be.

The stages of change model

The stages of change model proposes that when trying to change a behaviour we go through different stages (Figure 7.2). It is also known as the transtheoretical model of health behaviour change and is a very useful model as it focuses on the individual. It has been used in health interventions such as smoking cessation and weight loss.

The six stages in the model are listed under the following headings.

1. Precontemplation: not considering any changes

In this stage, using Case Study 7.4, Sarah has not even thought about giving up smoking. If she came into your pharmacy where you had a poster advertising smoking cessation support she might be oblivious to it. It is hard to identify people at this stage as they are not asking for help (and probably do not even know they might need it). All we can do is make our health promotion

FIGURE 7.2 **The stages of change model**

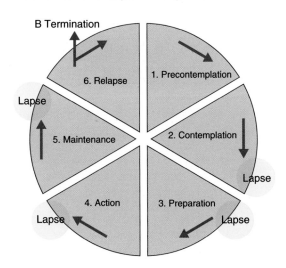

material as prominent as possible and wait. If a person makes an appointment in their general practice, or is receiving secondary care, we have a captive audience as the individual has become a patient for some reason. It is easier in this context to raise issues of health behaviour change although, of course, we cannot be sure that any suggestions will be taken up.

2. Contemplation: considering a change in behaviour

In this stage the idea of making changes is actually in a person's conscious thought. Sarah might have actually listened to her parents' fears for her health and decided that the holiday is more important. She might come into your community pharmacy and make a direct approach by saying: 'I'm thinking of giving up smoking', or she might pick up a smoking cessation leaflet while browsing and you might notice and ask: 'Are you thinking of giving up smoking?' Whatever the reason behind a person contemplating a change, you will need to be observant and tactful.

You need to be particularly tactful when communicating with someone about their weight. If someone comes in to your pharmacy and says they want to lose some weight there are ways of agreeing that you should use that do not offend. This is why you need to understand how our bodies work and how our behaviour is important in keeping us healthy—in other words understanding medicines use in the context of the individual.

3. Preparation: preparing to make changes

If Sarah was at this stage then she might have taken the advice of her pharmacist and decided to give up smoking. She might have chosen a date she is going to give up on and have told her parents so that they can support her.

4. Action: engaging in a new behaviour

Now we get to the scary part of actually making those changes. If you have ever tried to make such changes you will know that Sarah will be feeling a sense of anticipation as the chosen time comes nearer. She may feel enthusiastic about the changes she is about to make but she will also be experiencing a sense of fear that she may not have the willpower to succeed.

5. Maintenance: maintaining the behaviour change

The next stage in this cycle is keeping up that behaviour change and that is sometimes the hardest part. Because our behaviour is closely related to how we feel and what is going on in our lives we often use things that are bad for us to help us cope. During the maintenance stage it is important that people are given lots of support to enable them to believe in themselves and know that they can do it.

6. Relapse: returning to older/previous behaviours

Sometimes we just cannot cope, for whatever reason, and revert to our old behaviours. This is a normal part of health behaviour and people will often go round the cycle several times before actually succeeding.

As a pharmacist it is important that you too accept that people do not succeed in changing their behaviour the first time they try. If you do accept this then you can be supportive and encouraging so that people do not feel they have failed. A sense of failure can make it hard for people to bother to try again because they come to believe that they cannot succeed.

How effective is the stages of change model?

Having looked at the stages of change model there are some things that you need to consider about how effective it is in explaining health behaviour. Here are some problems with it:

- Matching the stage of the individual to the type of intervention is important. Identifying where people are in the cycle can be difficult, especially at the precontemplation stage. How do we know something that the patient does not even know herself?

- Individual rather than a population focus. The model helps us to design interventions that can be used on a one-to-one basis, but it does not explain how we can design interventions that will work for whole populations. Providing help on a one-to-one basis can be costly in financial terms and is time-consuming.

- Is there enough emphasis on the social aspects and meaning of the target behaviour? We do not live in a vacuum and most of our behaviour is influenced by other people in some way. The model does not include these wider social aspects of health behaviour and that is an important flaw.

Some of the other criticisms of the stages of change model are that we have no real evidence that behaviour change actually happens in stages. If you look back at the HBM you will remember that in that model there were 'cues to action' that prompted people to change their behaviour very quickly. It is possible that a person might go through all the changes in a very short space of time and that the process is too fast to make the stages important. For example, someone may move from precontemplation to action quickly (possibly as a result of a trigger or individual differences). Other key questions are:

- What prompts individuals to move from one stage to another?

- Does the fact that we have tried before make a difference?

- Is the model any better than asking someone if they have any plans to change their behaviour?

These are all good questions to think about and you should be questioning how the models explain health behaviour. We cannot answer these questions here, but you will find further reading at the end of the chapter if you want to learn more.

SELF CHECK 7.2

How would you identify that someone was at the preparation stage of making changes to their health behaviour? If someone came into your pharmacy and said they wanted to lose weight how would you support them in a pharmacy setting? Thinking about your own experiences can help you to understand how other people might feel.

SELF CHECK 7.3

How would you support the same person from Self Check 7.2 when they were in the action stage?

7.5 Measuring health and health inequalities

It is all very well talking about health behaviour and how models of behaviour can help us to understand why people do what they do, but why do we as health care professionals want to know these things? Whatever you feel about the models you have read about in this chapter I hope you have come to this conclusion: if we can learn how to predict which people might be susceptible to illness that results from health behaviour then we might be able to help them change their behaviour and give them the chance to be healthier.

Having models that help to explain health behaviour is only the first step in applying psychological theory to real-life practice. One of the major challenges which faces all of us who are interested in health care studies is the issue of how to measure health. As we saw in Section 7.2, all individuals are different and do not just conform to convenient models of behaviour. There will always be exceptions to the patterns of health behaviour that we see and so we need to find ways of measuring health. In Chapter 4 we looked at public health; one of the concerns of public health experts is that all people should be given the same opportunities to maintain the best possible health they can. To achieve this governments work hard to ensure that all people have access to health care and that people are not denied health care for reasons of, for example, sex, age, or ethnic origin. Health care planners and providers need to be constantly vigilant for the potential of inequality in health.

 Go back to Chapter 4 and refresh your knowledge if you need to.

Epidemiology

To help us to understand health psychology we need to know about the situations in which health and illness exist. This means that we need to use **epidemiology** to find ways of measuring how many people in different populations have specific conditions or diseases, whether these are transmitted from one person to another, and how this might happen. Epidemiologists look at patterns of disease and injury in groups of people or 'populations' and then try to find out why some groups of people develop illnesses more or less often than others. Some useful terms that

you will come across when studying epidemiology are given in Box 7.1.

This section is concluded by looking at two areas where we have to pay special attention to certain groups in the population and can lead to health inequalities. These differences are important to the practice of pharmacy and you might like to bear them in mind as you go through your studies.

Sex differences in health

As we know, men and women are different! And because of the differences in the way we are built we

BOX 7.1

Useful terms in epidemiology

- *Prevalence*: The number of cases of a disease or injury. This includes both previously reported and new cases at a particular time. For example, you might see reported that the number of cases of hay fever increased by 50% at the end of July.

- *Incidence*: This is similar to prevalence but it refers to new cases only. Here we might look at the incidence of influenza during a particular period of time.

- *Mortality*: This refers to death, usually on a large scale. It is usually described as the number of deaths per 1000 population in 1 year.

- *Morbidity*: This refers to poor health, injury, or disability of any cause and it is a term you will come across a lot in pharmacy practice. For example, on a patient's medication records you might read that they have comorbidities; this means that they have more than one thing wrong with them. Conditions such as diabetes and heart disease sometimes go together. In epidemiology, morbidity can refer to either the prevalence rate or the incidence rate.

- *Epidemic*: This refers to when the incidence of a disease increases very quickly.

- *Pandemic*: An epidemic that has spread across large regions (for example, continents) and can be worldwide.

'Gender' and 'sex'

You will often see the terms 'gender' and 'sex' used in the literature. There has been much debate about the use of these terms, with the feminist movement of the 1970s embracing the difference between the physical sex of a person and the 'social construction' of gender. For the purposes of this chapter we will use the term 'sex' because we are talking about physical differences between men and women.

To read more about this issue visit the World Health Organization website and search 'What do we mean by "sex" and "gender"?'

are prone to different diseases that are peculiar to our sex (see Box 7.2). For example, only women can develop cancer of the cervix because only women have a cervix. Similarly, only men can develop cancer of the prostate because only men have prostate glands.

Sometimes, the fact that a disease is more prevalent among women or men can lead to inequalities, as more emphasis is placed on one than the other. For example, efforts to find cures and treatments for cervical cancer have always been more prominent than efforts to fight prostate cancer. This may be because there has been greater publicity about cervical cancer, which has brought it more attention. This greater level of publicity might in itself create inequalities as it draws attention to one more than the other, with the result that one might be given more resources. A further difference this creates is that the more a condition is brought into the open and discussed, and the more high-profile people who are happy to talk about their experiences of the condition, the easier it becomes for

people to seek help at an earlier time and thus their chances of survival are increased. As a pharmacist you can publicize screening through posters and leaflets. This might encourage people to ask for more information and you can signpost them to the appropriate health care professional to obtain more help.

Ethnic differences in health

There are differences in the prevalence of diseases, and in the ways disease is perceived by people, in different parts of the world. These differences might be caused by genetic factors, making individuals more likely to develop conditions such as heart disease or forms of cancer. For example, sickle cell trait is a condition that affects red blood cells. Anyone can have sickle cell trait but it is most common in people whose family origin is Black African, Black Caribbean, or Black British.

 See Chapter 9 in **Therapeutics and Human Physiology** within this series for more information.

There are also some behavioural differences that are important. Some groups in society are less likely to seek help from a physician then others. This may be because disease is seen as something unacceptable or it might be that intimate examination is not possible for cultural reasons. Research conducted by Sheikh and Furman (2000) found that there was an association between cultural beliefs and whether or not people with mental health problems sought psychological help. Whatever the reasons, it is important to be aware that in a community pharmacy you may be an acceptable face of health care for some people and so you are in a position to help those who might be reluctant to seek help from a doctor.

7.6 Illness behaviour and the rights and obligations of patients and health care professionals

Wherever people come from, whatever their age, gender, race, culture, disability, or personal preferences,

they are all entitled to be treated in the same way. They also have the right to refuse treatment, and that right must be respected by health care professionals. However, in order for a patient to be able to decide whether they want to receive treatment or not they must have sufficient capacity to make the decision and have access to the appropriate information concerning their condition and treatment. It is the pharmacist's duty to support the patient in their decision-making by providing the information in a form accessible by the patient.

Under the terms of the Mental Capacity Act 2005, all adults are presumed to have sufficient mental capacity to decide whether or not to give their consent to treatment unless there is strong evidence to the contrary. If a person is deemed to have the mental capacity to make such decisions then they must be respected, even if going without treatment might lead to their death. This can be very hard for health care professionals to deal with, as knowing that there is a treatment available that has been rejected goes against the point of health care, which is to make people better and alleviate suffering.

The issue of a person's right to decide to accept treatment or not is an important one when exploring human behaviour. People have beliefs about illness and health that can be difficult to understand; an awareness of health psychology can contribute to this understanding and ensure that we take a holistic approach to pharmacy practice. Learning to be a pharmacist is not all about the science of medicines. No matter how extensive your knowledge of pharmacy practice and medicines use, if a person has decided they do not want to take a particular medicine then they have the right to this decision. All you can do at this point is try to understand why and provide support without being judgemental (see Case Study 7.5).

KEY POINT

You must respect a person's right to refuse treatment if they choose to do so, provided they have the mental capacity to make that decision. This is particularly relevant in medicines use as some people may make the decision that they do not want to take a medicine.

KEY POINT

The ability to provide patients and the public with expert, accurate advice should be based on evidence that you have obtained about particular medicines. This evidence should in turn be based on the results of research and we end this chapter by looking at the place of research in pharmacy practice.

129

CASE STUDY 7.5

James is 32 years of age, has always kept himself fit, and is the right weight for his height, although sometimes finds it hard to get enough exercise as his job means he spends a lot of time sitting down. James's father died at the age of 38 from a heart attack and was found to have had extensive coronary artery disease. James's doctor has told him that this family history means that he too may be at risk of developing coronary heart disease and has advised him to take statins. These are medicines that help to reduce blood cholesterol, a high level of which is a contributing factor to coronary heart disease and strokes.

James knows that he is at risk but also knows that if he goes on statins now he will have to take them for the rest of his life. James decides not to follow his doctor's advice and declines to take the statins.

REFLECTION QUESTIONS

1. What do you think about James's decision and what factors might he have taken into consideration in reaching that decision?

2. If James came into your pharmacy and asked your advice about whether or not he should take the statins what advice would you give him?

We are not going to give you the answers to these questions because your own beliefs as a health care professional are important and may change as you grow in your understanding of what it is to be a pharmacist.

Answer

7.7 **Behavioural and social sciences and their contribution to pharmacy practice research**

The behavioural and social sciences have also had an impact on the way pharmacy practice research is conducted. This section describes the importance of research and evidence-based practice.

Why is research important?

Learning to be a pharmacist takes a lot of time and effort. You need to know about the anatomy and physiology of the human body, the development of drugs, and how these act on the systems of the body. You will all have had some experience of how pharmaceutical scientists develop medicines and that they conduct research both to design medicines that target particular conditions and to work out the best way they can be delivered into the body.

As a pharmacist your job is to ensure that people take their medicines safely and effectively (if they want to), and so research is also carried out into what the job of a pharmacist is and how they do it. This is called pharmacy practice research.

Pharmacists do not work in isolation from other health care professionals. They work as part of a multidisciplinary team to deliver the best care possible to patients. Each member of a multidisciplinary team brings specialist skills to patient care that the others do not possess. The success of teams depends on individuals knowing where their expertise ends and another's begins. We must be aware of our own competence and work within it, ensuring that we admit when we do not know something. Knowing these things and being able to reflect on them is all part of being a professional pharmacist. In the same way that health care professionals work together and learn from each other in their daily practice, they also work together to undertake research.

Evidence-based practice

Health care must be based on sound evidence from research. Incorporating the findings of research into the delivery of care to patients is called evidence-based practice. All schools of pharmacy should be committed to developing the skills of students to ensure that they go into their future careers as competent, confident health care professionals—fully equipped to meet the demands of their profession. This includes the ability to evaluate evidence and relate it to practice. The mindset or attitude of the student is very important to personal development. How you perceive research, and the importance you ascribe to its application in practice, will determine the advice you give to patients and other health care professionals. You should be developing a positive approach to research and its applications in practice alongside the development of your other knowledge and skills. Using evidence to support your decision-making with regards to medicines contributes to your competence as a pharmacist.

Methodological rigour

When reading of health research in a journal, for example about a particular medicine, there are several questions worth considering:

- How do you know that what you are reading is true?
- How do you know that the research that it is based on was done properly?
- How do you know whether it is relevant to your area of pharmacy?

In your practice as a pharmacist, in whatever setting, you are going to be called upon to provide people with advice about medicines. For example, if you are on a hospital ward round with a doctor and other members of the health care team you may be asked which of two particular drugs you would recommend for a patient. The advice you give *must* be based on your knowledge and skills as a pharmacist and your understanding of the very latest research into those drugs, as well as your knowledge of how people's beliefs affect their health behaviour. Your decision will therefore be evidence-based and may make the difference between life and death for some patients.

SELF CHECK 7.4

How might you go about answering a prescriber who asks whether one medicine is safer than another medicine?

Being able to critically appraise research is one of the things you will learn as you progress with your degree, and will equip you with the skills to give good advice. This will allow you to appreciate the strengths and weaknesses of a particular study.

Social science research methods

In this chapter we have focused on how the behavioural sciences can contribute to pharmacy practice. If we have a question that we want to answer using research then this must be carried out in a way that gives both accurate and useful answers. This is called the **research method**, and the method we choose will probably have come from the behavioural and social sciences which pioneered many of the research methods now used by the health sciences.

There are two main research methodologies:

1. *Quantitative research*: enables us to get answers from large numbers of people, which we can analyse using statistics and compare the results. One of the ways to obtain data is using a questionnaire with set responses. This limits what can be asked (for example, Do you smoke? Answer: yes or no.)

2. *Qualitative research*: is better for smaller sample sizes. Descriptive information (rather than mathematical data) is collected using questionnaires with open questions or by conducting interviews. To find out why people do what they do it is sometimes better to ask them with an open question (for example, Why do you smoke? Explain your answer fully.).

We would use quantitative methods to find out whether people had been diagnosed with cancer, what type of cancer, when they were diagnosed, and how they were treated. However, we could then use qualitative methods to interview some of those people and find out from them what it was like to experience a diagnosis and treatment of cancer—in other words, what did it *feel* like from their perspective?

When you come to do research do not be afraid to look at other disciplines and use their methods in your own study. Pharmacy practice has been doing this for some time and most research can be conducted in similar ways, with the only difference being the subject matter. As far as pharmacy practice is concerned, we can explore the role of pharmacists in the delivery of health care and compare it with the role of doctors, nurses, and other professions. What you learn from each other in practice and research can not only enrich your knowledge and understanding of pharmacy but also make you a better pharmacist.

➤ This chapter described the behavioural and social sciences and how an understanding of these might contribute to the pharmacist's provision of health care.

➤ It looked at definitions of health and illness.

➤ It focused on theories from health psychology and how these might help us to understand why people do the things they do in terms of their health.

➤ It looked at health measurement and health inequalities and the rights of patients.

➤ Finally, the chapter explored research methods in social science and how these might be used by pharmacists.

Berry, D. *Risk, Communication and Health Psychology*. Open University Press, 2004.

> This book gives a good overview of the importance of communication in the provision of health care.

Breakwell, G.M., Hammond, S., Fife-Schaw, C., and Smith, J.A. (Eds). *Research Methods in Psychology*. 3rd edn. Sage, 2006.

> This is an excellent book which provides guidance on the many research methods available to researchers in all disciplines.

Cameron, L. and Leventhal, H. (Eds). *The Self-Regulation of Health and Illness Behaviour*. Routledge, 2003.

> This book gives more details about health and illness behaviour.

Ogden, J. *Health Psychology: A Textbook*. 4th edn. Open University Press, 2007.

> Just one of many textbooks on health psychology.

Taylor, D., Bury, M., Campling, N.A., Carter, S., Garfied, S., Newbould, J., and Rennie, T. *Review of the use of the Health Belief Model (HBM), the Theory of Reasoned Action (TRA), the Theory of Planned Behaviour (TPB) and the Trans-Theoretical Model (TTM) to Study and Predict Health Related Behaviour Change*. School of Pharmacy, University of London, 2007.

> A good text if you want to understand more about the theories of health behaviour and how these relate to behaviour change.

Bonita, R., Beaglehole, R., and Kjellstrom, T. *Basic Epidemiology*. 2nd edn. World Health Organization, 2006.

> This is a good text for those new to epidemiology.

Pharmaceutical care

8

JASON HALL

Pharmacists are key members of the health care team. This chapter seeks to illustrate how pharmacists can make a positive contribution to patient care. It will introduce the factors that should be considered when deciding which treatment option is most appropriate. It will describe the issues pharmacists should explore when reviewing medicine use with patients, and will provide an example of a systematic approach to identifying pharmaceutical care issues. It will also integrate material covered in the previous chapters of the book.

Learning objectives

Having read this chapter you are expected to be able to:

➤ Introduce the factors to consider when comparing different treatment options.

➤ Appreciate that treatment options can be compared by considering the effectiveness, safety, cost, and patient acceptability of the different options.

➤ Define pharmaceutical care.

➤ Develop a systematic approach to reviewing how patients use their medication.

➤ Identify the range of issues to be explored with patients when discussing their medication.

➤ Review how the range of pharmaceutical services might evolve and consider the impact of this evolution on pharmacy's future professional status.

8.1 Which medication is most appropriate?

When patients receive a medicine they expect that it will be the most suitable one for them. How does a prescriber know which medicine is most suitable for a particular patient? The prescriber could base the decision on their experience and use what has worked well in the past. Obviously, such a method of selection is not helpful for those starting out on their career. It is also not a very scientific approach

either, as prescribers may have seen relatively small numbers of patients with a particular condition and so there will have been no attempt to compare the results in a fair and scientific manner. It would be much more reliable to base decisions on data derived from several thousand patients who have been treated in a standard manner which allows results to be compared.

It has been suggested that the quality of prescribing should be assessed against four aims, which are to:

- Maximize effectiveness
- Minimize harm
- Minimize cost
- Respect patient choice.

Using each of these four aims of good prescribing we will now consider how patient data can be compared in a robust way to generate useful evidence about medicines.

Maximizing effectiveness

The term 'placebo effect' is used to describe the situation when a patient responds to a medicine that contains no active ingredient (a placebo). When a new medicine is tested, half of the test population is given the medicine with the active ingredient (the drug) and the other half is given a placebo. This is done blind, which means that those taking part in the study do not know whether they have taken the drug or the placebo. To reduce the risk of bias, trials are frequently double blinded: neither the patients nor the health care staff administering the medication know who has taken which preparation. All medicines licensed for use in the UK must have shown benefit compared with a placebo.

Manufacturers of new medicines do not have to demonstrate benefit against similar products on the market. The existence of a market authorization or a product licence does not indicate how good a medicine is. To assess this, we need to review the evidence. Evidence comes from a variety of different sources and there are huge differences between the quality and reliability of these.

Clinical trials

Clinical trials provide a great deal of the evidence on how effective a medicine is. When reviewing this evidence we need to consider:

- The number of patients included in the trail; the larger the sample the better. When only a small sample is used the analysis of the data can be skewed by a few unusual occurrences.

- The location of the trial. The greater the number of locations used the less likely the study is to be affected by local factors.

- The similarity of the population sample to the patients we are treating. Did the trial include males and females? Were ethnic minorities included? What was the age range of the sample? Clinical trials do not always include the same proportions of different groups of patients as you may see in the patient populations that you serve.

- Was the trial blinded or double blinded?

- Did the trial compare against a placebo or similar medicines? If it compared against similar medicines were comparable dosages used? There is no point saying drug A was more effective than drug B if the dose of drug A was much higher than that of drug B.

- Was the trial sponsored by the pharmaceutical industry? There is a risk of bias to show a particular drug is effective if the manufacturer of that drug has funded the study. However, many high-quality studies are funded by the industry, so industry sponsorship does not always equate to bias.

- What was the endpoint of the study? Ideally, the end point of the study should be the same as the objective you are trying to achieve for the patient. However, there are trials where it would not be ethical to use the actual desired end point. For example, there is good evidence that statins reduce cholesterol and lower the risk of heart attacks and ischaemic strokes. The desired outcome of statin therapy is to reduce the risk of adverse cardiovascular events. However, if a new statin were developed it is likely that the clinical trials would investigate its ability to lower cholesterol (which can be assessed easily in a relatively short period of time) rather than its ability to prevent heart attacks and ischaemic strokes because it would be unethical to measure the number of heart attacks and strokes in a group of patients when there is proven treatment available.

Researchers can also compare the results of several clinical trials in a **meta-analysis**, which involves statistically combining the results of several clinical trials. The results from such an analysis are much more reliable because the numbers tend to be larger and there is less risk of bias, as many different researchers have been involved. Meta-analyses are said to be the gold standard in evidence.

Minimizing harm

All medicines have the potential to harm patients (see Box 8.1) but the risk is not the same for all medicines or all patients. Clinical trials and systematic reviews will also address the safety of the medicines under review. The points to consider when assessing the quality of evidence from clinical trials and systematic reviews described under 'Maximizing effectiveness' in this section apply equally to assessing the likelihood of a medicine to cause harm (number of participants, blinded or double blinded, sponsored by the pharmaceutical industry, etc.).

The data on the safety of a medicine obtained from Phase III clinical trials are very useful. However, these data are limited and there are a number of reasons why. The patients who have been included in these clinical trials may not be representative of the patients that you are likely to come across in practice, as they are unlikely to have the same comorbidities or to be taking the same range of other medications. The volume of safety data on the medicine is limited owing to the relatively low numbers of patients who have taken the medicine during the clinical trials. The medicine may have been taken by a few hundred or a few thousand patients, but harmful effects that are very rare may not have been detected.

 See Chapter 1 for a reminder about the different phases in clinical trials.

It is therefore necessary to have ongoing monitoring of a medicine's safety to detect harmful effects as hundreds of thousands of patients take the medicine. **Pharmacovigilance** is the term used to describe the ongoing monitoring of a medicine's safety, the assessment of risk, and informing health professionals and patients regarding a medicine's safety. The safety of all medicines, including over-the-counter and herbal remedies, is monitored via the yellow card system, whereby health professionals report suspected ADRs by completing a yellow form that can be found at the back of the *British National Formulary* (*BNF*). All ADRs to new medicines (which can be identified by the presence of a black triangle next to the medicine's name in the *BNF* monograph) should be reported. For established medicines it is necessary to report serious ADRs, such as those which are incapacitating, disabling, or life threatening, or those which result in prolonged hospital admission or death of the patient.

For some medicines the risk of harm is much higher than for others. Adverse effects are unwanted effects that occur when medicines are taken at the recommended dosage. Side effects are effects that a drug may have which are secondary to the main effect and may be beneficial or harmful. The *BNF* reports the frequency of side effects of drugs using the following terms:

- *Very common*: greater than 1 in 10
- *Common*: between 1 in 10 and 1 in 100
- *Less common*: between 1 in 100 and 1 in 1000
- *Rare*: between 1 in 1000 and 1 in 10 000
- *Very rare*: less than 1 in 10 000.

For example, some of the side effects listed in the *BNF* for glyceryl trinitrate include:

- Postural hypotension
- Throbbing headache
- Dizziness

BOX 8.1

The importance of minimizing adverse drug reactions

Improving health care outcomes

In 2004 a study reported that 6.5% of all the admissions to two National Health Service (NHS) hospitals were owing to adverse drug reactions (ADRs). Of those admitted, 80% were directly because of the ADR, with the other 20% being admitted for other reasons but where ADR could have been a contributing factor.

Maximizing efficiency

The projected annual cost to the NHS from admissions associated with ADR has been calculated to be £466 million.

Less commonly:

- Nausea, vomiting
- Heartburn
- Flushing

Very rarely:

- Angle closure glaucoma.

Note that the *BNF* does not provide any indication regarding the frequency of the first three side effects in the above list. In such cases the frequency should be assumed to be common or very common.

Information on the frequency of side effects, such as that provided by the *BNF*, is very useful but it is rarely sufficiently detailed to permit a comparison of safety between different medicines. In many cases the *BNF* presents the side effects of all drugs within a class together at the beginning of that subsection rather than under each individual drug monograph; for example, the majority of the side effects of statins are listed together. There are some sections where the *BNF* provides greater detail on the safety of drugs. The section on non-steroidal anti-inflammatory drugs (NSAIDs) provides a comparison of the risk of gastro-intestinal side effects for a range of NSAIDs. It also advises that the risks are greater for elderly patients and recommends no more than one NSAID is used at a time.

Some patients are more likely to suffer harm when taking medicines. There are many ways in which a drug can cause harm but the risk of harm tends to increase with factors that influence the level of drug in the body. The rate at which the body eliminates the drug is often the most important factor. Patients with kidney failure or liver failure will have reduced elimination of the drug and are more at risk of experiencing an adverse drug reaction. Renal and hepatic function decrease during the aging process so that elderly patients eliminate drugs more slowly than younger patients. Patients taking several drugs are also at greater risk of experiencing an adverse drug reaction.

Minimizing cost

All medicines have a cost associated with their use and somebody must pay these costs. Costs may be paid for by the patient, the state, or an insurance company. No one wants to pay more than they have to so there is a desire to keep costs to a minimum, yet have a maximum benefit. In the case of the state, it wants to keep costs low either to reduce the tax burden on society or to allow a greater proportion of the population to be treated. When there are different treatment options there are likely to be a range of costs associated with each option. All factors must be taken into account when considering the costs and benefits of these different options. This is known as cost–benefit analysis. For example, a medicine that costs more initially may turn out to cost less in the long term if there are lower rates of relapse or fewer adverse effects that would also require medications or hospitalizations (see Box 8.2 for a worked example).

To allow a fair comparison of cost–benefit ratios for different medicines we need to be able to measure the benefits and harm associated with the different medicines. The benefits of some medicines are relatively obvious and easy to measure, such as preventing death or reducing length of hospital stay. There are many other conditions where the benefits may be less tangible and more difficult to measure, and objective assessments of a patient's quality of life have been developed. Some of these are disease specific; one example is the Arthritis Impact Measurement Scale (AIMS), which provides a score for a patient based upon their mobility, ability to perform physical and household activities, dexterity, pain, and depression. The scores before and after treatment can be compared to provide an objective measure of how well a medicine is able to treat a condition. There are also 'generic' assessments which are not related to any particular condition. They can measure the impact of a condition and treatment on a patient's quality of life. The SF36 is one of a number of questionnaires that assess the patient's physical and mental health.

More often than not, funding for health care treatments is limited and difficult decisions need to be made concerning which conditions can be treated by the health care funding body. The funding body may wish to compare a range of different treatments to determine which produce the greatest benefit before deciding what it will fund. Data from clinical trials and quality of life assessments can be combined to produce the **quality-adjusted life year (QALY)**. One QALY is

BOX 8.2

Cost–benefit comparison for three different medicines

Treatment options

- **Option 1**: Medicine A costs £10.00 for 28 tablets; the dose is one tablet each day. Ten per cent of patients develop gastrointestinal discomfort requiring the co-prescribing of medicine X to protect the stomach. Medicine X costs £12.00 for 28 tablets (dose: one tablet daily).

- **Option 2**: Medicine B costs £15.00 for 56 tablets; the dose is two tablets each day. Five per cent of patients develop a skin rash during initiation of the treatment, which requires the co-prescribing of medicine Y for 4 weeks until the rash subsides. Medicine Y costs £8.00 per 28 tablets (dose: one tablet two times a day).

- **Option 3**: Medicine C costs £13.00 for 28 tablets; the dose is one tablet each day. Twelve per cent of patients develop diarrhoea during the first month, which requires the co-prescribing of medicine Z for 1 week. Medicine Z costs £5.00 for 28 tablets (dose: one tablet four times a day).

Treatment costs

How much would it cost to treat 100 patients for 1 year (52 weeks)?

Option 1: Medicine A: A pack of 28 tablets lasts 4 weeks, so for the whole year each patient would need 13 packs. For all 100 patients that gives a total number of 1300 packs.

Number of packs needed × price of each pack = total cost

$$1300 \times £10 = £13000$$

Medicine X: A pack of 28 tablets lasts 4 weeks, so for the whole year each patient would need 13 packs. Only ten of the patients need it, so that gives a total number of 130 packs.

$$130 \times £12 = £1560$$

The following equation can also be used for the calculation:

$$\left(\left(\frac{\text{Cost of pack}}{\text{Weeks the pack lasts}} \right) \times \text{Weeks the medication is to be taken} \right) \times \text{No. of patients}$$

$$((10.00 \times 52)/4) \times 100 = £13000 \text{ for medicine A}$$

$$((12.00 \times 52)/4) \times 10 = £1560 \text{ for medicine X}$$

Total = £14 560

Option 2:

$$((15.00 \times 52)/4) \times 100 = £19500 \text{ for medicine B}$$

$$((16.00 \times 4)/4) \times 5 = £80 \text{ for medicine Y}$$

Total = £19 580

Option 3:

$$((13 \times 52)/4) \times 100 = £16900 \text{ for medicine C}$$

$$((5 \times 1)/4) \times 12 = £15 \text{ for medicine Z}$$

Total = £16 915

equal to one year in 'perfect health' for one patient. The QALY can be used to compare the cost benefit of different medical treatments. Typically, the number of additional QALYs per treatment can be compared for a range of treatments (see Box 8.3).

Respecting patient choice

Pharmacists should explore the patient's orientation towards medicines. Some patients may not wish to be treated with any medicines and it is important that we establish this and respect their views. Concordance involves the health care practitioner and patient discussing and agreeing, as equals, what course of action should be taken.

 See Section 5.10 'Giving the medicine to the patient', in Chapter 5, for examples of adherence, and Section 6.7 'Communication with patients: the development of the art of consultation', in Chapter 6, for more in-depth discussion on developing consultation skills.

The quality-adjusted life year (QALY)

The average survival time for patients with a particular medical condition is 4 years and their health is assessed as being 50% of perfect health (quality of life = 0.5).

Number of QALYs: $4 \times 0.5 = 2$

Two medicines are available to treat the condition. Medicine P increases average survival time to 10 years but does not have any impact on quality of life, which remains at 50% for those with the condition. Medicine Q increases survival time to 8 years and improves quality of life such that the patients are assessed as having 75% of perfect health.

Number of QALYs for medicine P: $10 \times 0.5 = 5$

Number of additional QALYs for P: $5 - 2 = 3$

Number of QALYs for medicine Q: $8 \times 0.75 = 6$

Number of additional QALYs for Q: $6 - 2 = 4$

Medicine P produces an additional three QALYs whereas medicine Q produces an additional four QALYs.

Some medicines may be more pleasant to use owing to taste, solubility, or frequency of administration. Medical devices such as inhalers make certain medicines easier to take, and even the packaging of a medicine can improve a patient's concordance because less bulky packaging makes it easier for patients to carry their medicine with them when they go out. Pharmacists should discuss with patients how easy they find it to take or use their medication. If a medicine needs to be taken four times a day and the patient frequently forgets one or more of their doses then the pharmacist can offer advice about dosage aids such as a 'dosette' box. The easier it is for a patient to take a medicine the more likely they are to use it as prescribed.

However, those that are easier are also frequently more expensive. A patient could have one 25 mg diclofenac sodium tablet three times a day or they could have one 75 mg diclofenac sodium modified release (MR) tablet once a day. Both the 25 mg × 3 and the 75 mg MR should have a similar therapeutic effect, but the MR formulation is up to five times the cost of the 25 mg tablet. One approach is to consider the impact on adherence and to restrict those expensive medicines which are easier to take to those patients for whom an alternative would affect compliance. It is important that patients are involved in this review and assessment of medical treatment because different patients may want different things from their treatment. For some patients, preventing progression of a condition may be the priority whereas for others it may be controlling the symptoms.

Patients may have difficulty with a drug or formulation or they may be unwilling to take certain medicines. For example, a patient may not be willing to take medicines that are derived from animal products, such as those containing gelatine. In addition, the patient's lifestyle may make taking a particular medicine more difficult. Medicines which cause drowsiness would be more difficult to take for a patient who drives or operates machinery as part of their livelihood.

Accessing evidence in practice

Deciding which medication is the most appropriate is often not an easy decision. One medicine that is more effective than another may not be as safe, may be expensive, or may be unpleasant to take so that patients dislike it. There is frequently a trade-off between these four parameters.

The term evidence-based medicine has been used to describe the process of systematically finding, appraising, and using contemporaneous research findings as the basis for clinical decisions. Its approach allows the results from many studies to be fairly compared and used to help inform clinical decisions (see Box 8.4 for a list of the different steps involved in evidence-based medicine).

There are a great many different references and sources of information on medicines available to

Four steps in evidence-based medicine

1. Formulate a clear clinical question from a patient's problem.

2. Search the literature for relevant clinical articles.

3. Evaluate (critically appraise) the evidence for its validity and usefulness.

4. Implement useful findings in clinical practice.

support pharmacists in their review of medication. Consideration must be made regarding the reliability of the source. Questions to consider include:

- Who is the publisher?
- Is the article sponsored by the pharmaceutical industry or some other group with a vested interest which could suggest bias?
- When was it published?

Clinical guidelines have been published for some conditions. Organizations such as NICE (National Institute for Health and Clinical Excellence), SIGN (Scottish Intercollegiate Guidelines Network) and many trusts publish clinical guidelines to support practice. Clinical guidelines can help guide prescribers by directing them towards which questions to ask and which tests to perform. They also support decision-making by recommending treatments. These recommendations are ideally based upon the best available evidence; however, if evidence is lacking then they may be based upon expert opinion. All guidelines should clearly state whether they are evidence-based or expert opinion-based. Prescribers can choose not to follow a clinical guideline but if they do then they must be able to justify why they have followed a different course of action.

 See 'Prescribing decision-making' in Section 5.3 of Chapter 5 for an example.

Formularies were some of the earliest sources of information on medicines; they were originally reference works which contained recipes or, more correctly, the formulae of medicines, which allowed pharmacists to prepare the medicine extemporaneously. The formulae have now disappeared such that formularies are now lists of medicines. The *BNF* is the best known and most widely used in the UK. Some trusts and general practices have introduced a formulary for local use. There is not always a clear distinction between formularies and guidelines because many formularies contain some guidance on which medicine to use in which situation, and some guidelines even name specific drugs to be used in specific circumstances.

> **KEY POINT**
>
> The evidence for benefit and harm must be reviewed, and the costs and patients' preferences must be considered, when selecting medicines.

8.2 **Pharmaceutical care**

Basing decisions upon the best available evidence is clearly a positive step, but it is also necessary to take the patient's personal circumstances into account. Pharmacists need to be able to determine which medicine is the most appropriate for a particular patient when they are recommending a medicine for over-the-counter sale or when reviewing the prescribing of another health care professional.

 See Chapter 5 for a discussion of clinical and legal perspectives to take into account when prescribing or recommending medicines for over-the-counter sale.

Legal and clinical checks should be performed each time a pharmacist dispenses a medicine or sells an over-the-counter medicine. However, these checks just tell us whether a medicine is suitable for a patient. They do not necessarily tell us whether it is the most appropriate medicine, whether the patient is actually responding, or whether they are suffering adverse effects. Some medicines do not work in all patients and some can cause unacceptable adverse effects.

Accepting responsibility and specifying outcomes

It is not always possible to predict who will benefit from a taking a medicine and who will suffer harm. There have been cases of patients taking medicines for many years without seeing any benefit and some even experiencing harm. The pharmaceutical care approach was proposed by Hepler and Strand (1990) to help ensure that medicine use leads to improvements in patient care. They defined pharmaceutical care as: 'The responsible provision of drug therapy for the purpose of achieving definite outcomes that improve a patient's quality of life.' The key words in this definition are 'responsible' and 'outcomes':

- Who will take *responsibility* for pharmaceutical care: that patients receive the most appropriate medicines, resulting in improvements in health with minimal side effects?

  – As experts in drug formulation and drug use, pharmacists are in an ideal position to do this.

- We must be clear what the desired *outcome* is for all drug therapy. This may seem obvious but the reason for starting a medicine may not be documented in the patient's medical notes and the patient may not be aware why they are taking all their medications.

  – We should consider outcomes, such as controlling the patient's condition, and also managing any adverse effects associated with medicine use. Outcomes should be specific and measurable (for example, blood pressure 120/80 mmHg), observable (for example, elimination of skin rash), or reportable (for example, patient reports improvement in pain).

See Case Study 8.1 for examples of specifying desired outcomes for patients. If pharmacists take responsibility for monitoring and assessing whether specified outcomes have been achieved then the patient's quality of life should improve.

SELF CHECK 8.1

What are the therapeutic outcomes for the following patients? (a) Naina Patel, aged 54, who was diagnosed 3 years ago with type 2 diabetes mellitus. She is currently prescribed metformin 500 mg; (b) Suresh Shah, aged 52, who was diagnosed with angina 5 years ago. He is currently prescribed atenolol 50 mg and glyceryl trinitrate 500 μg.

KEY POINT

Pharmacists must be prepared to take responsibility for monitoring and achieving desired pharmaceutical outcomes.

Monitoring outcomes

Determining the clinical appropriateness of medication requires knowledge of physiology, biochemistry, pharmacology, and therapeutics. As many aspects of these topics are not covered until later in the MPharm programme, assessing the clinical appropriateness of medication is beyond the scope of this text book.

CASE STUDY 8.1

Specifying therapeutic outcomes

Mrs JT was diagnosed with rheumatoid arthritis (RA) 7 years ago. She tells you that she wants to be able to control the inflammation and pain to such a level that she is able to go out shopping on her own. She is prescribed diclofenac 75 mg modified release tablets, one to be taken twice a day.

REFLECTION QUESTION

What outcomes are you trying to achieve when prescribing Mrs JT with diclofenac 75 mg?

Answers

1 The therapeutic outcomes you are seeking are:
  - Manage the pain and inflammation due to RA.
  - Prevent progression of the RA.
2 The safety outcomes you are seeking are:
  - Minimize side effects.
  - Prevent adverse effects.
  - Prevent or manage drug interactions.

However, the principles that underpin this can be considered here.

Maximizing effectiveness

Not every medicine will work equally well in all patients. Some patients may not receive any benefit from a particular medicine. To ensure a medicine is effective in a patient we need to monitor the patient. In some cases this will be relatively straightforward and will involve asking the patient whether the symptoms have improved; for example, 'does this medicine control your pain?' In other cases we may need to perform tests such as measuring the patient's blood pressure to ensure that an antihypertensive medicine is working or taking a blood sample to check the levels of electrolytes or hormones. In a small number of cases we need to monitor the level of drug in the patient as part of **therapeutic drug monitoring (TDM)**. TDM is reserved for a relatively small number of medicines and patients. Lithium may require TDM because it has a narrow therapeutic window (the safe dose is very close to the toxic dose where adverse effects can occur). Patients on several medicines that could interact, or patients with renal or hepatic problems, may also require TDM.

If the desired outcome is not being fully met then the pharmacist should explore possible reasons:

- Is the patient receiving the appropriate drug for that indication?
- Is the patient able to take the drug appropriately?
- Can the patient afford the drug?
- Is the patient receiving enough of the drug?

Depending upon the responses to these questions it may be appropriate to change the dose or formulation of the drug, to change to a new medicine altogether, or to add an additional medicine.

Minimizing harm

Some adverse effects must be monitored via blood testing of the patient. Diuretics can upset the electrolyte balance in the body and blood testing is used to monitor this. The availability of electronic medical records allows patients in need of review to be identified.

Pharmacists also have an important role to play in monitoring any possible harmful effects resulting from the taking or using of medicines and should be alert to cautions and contraindications when they are reviewing a patient's therapy. It is important to speak to patients or their carers to explore whether they are suffering any side effects or adverse effects from the medicines. In some cases the pharmacist can help the patient to minimize the risk of side effects by explaining how a medicine should be used. For example, patients taking glyceryl trinitrate (GTN) sublingual (under the tongue) tablets to treat angina may suffer a throbbing headache. This headache can often be avoided by spitting the GTN tablet out as soon as the angina pain resolves.

Sometimes drugs interact with each other and this can have an effect on patients. It is important to realize that not all interactions are bad, but some can be. For example, many interactions involve changes to the enzymes involved in the metabolism of other drugs, leading to either increased toxicity or reduced effectiveness.

- Cimetidine, which is used to treat conditions caused by excessive amounts of acid being produced in the stomach, is known to inhibit the metabolism of some drugs. When it is given with phenytoin or theophylline it can lead to increased levels of the other drug and possible toxic effects.
- Carbamazepine, prescribed for epilepsy, is known to induce the production of certain enzymes, and when it is given with coumarins or ciclosporin it will accelerate their metabolism, leading to a reduced effect.

Once potential interactions have been detected there needs to be an assessment of the likelihood of harm. The *BNF* uses the black dot system whereby interactions which are likely to be clinically significant are annotated with a black dot. These interactions generally mean that alternative medicines should be selected first unless there is no alternative. If the drugs must be given then dosages may need to be altered and the clinical effects may need to be monitored more closely. Those without a black dot do not usually have serious consequences so no action is usually required. However, if there are other factors such as renal or hepatic impairment then an interaction without a black dot could become significant.

Patients taking multiple medicines, patients with renal or hepatic problems, and elderly patients are more likely to experience harm from medicines and extra care should be taken with these patients.

If the patient is experiencing unwanted effects then the pharmacist should explore possible causes:

- Is the drug having any undesired effects?
- Is the drug contraindicated?
- Is the drug one that should be used with caution?
- Is the patient taking a drug that is no longer indicated?
- Is there any inappropriate duplication of therapy?
- Is the patient taking *too much* of the correct drug.
- Are there any drugs which could interact?
- Are there any patient factors which could affect drug handling (for example, renal or hepatic problems)?

Depending upon the responses to these questions it may be appropriate to change the dose or formulation of the drug, to change to a new medicine altogether, or to add an additional medicine.

Minimizing cost

The costs of medicines change over time. When a drug is no longer covered by its patent it can be manufactured by other companies, who will produce cheaper generic versions. Reviewing a patient's medication can produce considerable savings if products can be switched to cheaper alternatives. It is important that any such changes are discussed with the patient to ensure the patient understands why the change is being made and also is fully assured that their care is not being compromised.

 See 'Respecting patient choice' in this section.

Pharmacists can review whether patients can afford all the medicines that they require and can offer advice to help minimize the cost. If the medicines are purchased over the counter the pharmacist could recommend cheaper alternatives or refer the patient to an NHS prescriber. If the medicine is prescribed on the NHS in England and the patient is not exempt from NHS prescription charges then the pharmacist could recommend a prepayment certificate. If the medicines are prescribed privately then the pharmacist could offer to speak to the prescriber to recommend a cheaper alternative.

It is also important to realize that the costs associated with medicine use are not just financial. Medicine use can also have emotional costs. Symptoms which are not controlled and adverse effects can have an impact on the patient, their carer, and their family. Patients may have to take time off work or engage a carer to look after their dependents.

Respecting patient choice

When patients are first diagnosed with a new condition they may be in some shock and may know very little about the condition. As time progresses they are likely to learn more about their condition and its management from professional sources and also from others such as friends, family, magazines, and the Internet. Some of this information may be reliable and some may be misleading, but as the patient's knowledge increases their views on how they wish to be treated may well change.

> **KEY POINT**
>
> It is very important that you do not assume what a patient's views on their medicines are. You must also understand and respect that patients' views about their treatments can change over time.

Scientific training combined with the development of patient-centred skills help pharmacists occupy a unique position in the health care team, as discussed in Chapter 1. Combining all these skills may appear to be a challenge, but improving the quality of medicines management can produce major improvements in patient care (see Case Study 8.2).

8.3 Medication review in practice

Pharmacists in primary and secondary care have an important role to play in reviewing medicines to ensure that all medicines (prescribed medicines and over-the-counter medicines) continue to be appropriate. There are different levels of medication review (see Figure 8.1).

Hospital pharmacists have been reviewing patients' medicines during ward rounds for many years. Their clinical knowledge and skills have been put to very good use. They have access to the patient and to the patient's medical history, making this a clinical medication review (Level 3). The patient's medical history contains details on previous consultations, symptoms, laboratory test results, prescribed medication, and diagnosis. It is possible to review how a condition has progressed and what treatments have been tried. Hospital pharmacists also have access to medical and nursing staff, which has been a very positive factor in the success of this role.

Pharmacists working in general practice have access to a patient's medical history and will also have access to the GP so they can also undertake clinical medication reviews. Community pharmacists do not currently have access to the patient's medical history and access to the GP may be more difficult, which limits their ability to become fully involved in this level of review. In many cases the conditions which the patient has been diagnosed with can only be determined by consulting the medical notes. Many drugs have more than one indication and patients may not always be aware of the indications. Monitoring some conditions can only be fully achieved with access to laboratory and test data. For example, blood tests are required to diagnose and to select appropriate treatment for patients with anaemia.

A number of initiatives have been introduced in the community to enhance patient understanding and use of medicines. The Medication Use Review (MUR) in England is an example of a service where pharmacists meet patients to discuss their use of medicines. This is not a full clinical review as pharmacists do not have access to the patient's medical notes, but it is a good opportunity to gather information on how the patient uses their prescribed and purchased medicines. The pharmacist can help them understand their medicines more fully and will also identify any medication problems and possible solutions. Case Study 8.2 outlines the components of a typical MUR and what can be gained from the review.

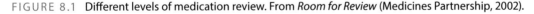

FIGURE 8.1 Different levels of medication review. From *Room for Review* (Medicines Partnership, 2002).

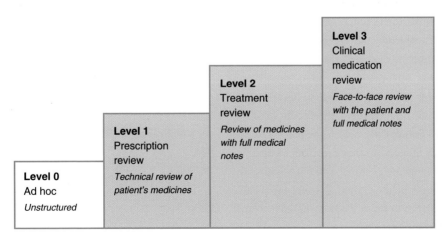

Level 0
Ad hoc
Unstructured

Level 1
Prescription review
Technical review of patient's medicines

Level 2
Treatment review
Review of medicines with full medical notes

Level 3
Clinical medication review
Face-to-face review with the patient and full medical notes

Preparing for a review

The following breakdown is an indication of the different aspects that a pharmacist can explore with a patient to help their understanding and use of medicines. To gain the maximum benefit from such a review it is important that the pharmacist is aware of all the medicines that the patient is taking. In community pharmacy the pharmacist can access the patient medication record (PMR), which will tell the pharmacist what the patient has been prescribed. It is important to note that this may not be a complete record as the patient may have visited another community pharmacist to have a prescription dispensed. There is also no certainty that the patient has actually been taking the medications that have been prescribed. In the hospital, the pharmacist should have access to the prescription chart for inpatients but this may not be available for outpatients or for patients who have just been admitted to the hospital. It is important that pharmacists in community pharmacy and in hospital ask the patient about any medications or herbal remedies that they have purchased over the counter.

Establishing how much patients know about their medications and how they are taking them is usually best achieved by speaking to the patient or their carer. It can help to determine if the patients know how and when they should be taking their medication. Patients may be more likely to take their medication at the appropriate times if they know why they are taking it. For example, many patients with asthma have repeat prescriptions for a salbutamol inhaler and a beclometasone inhaler. Salbutamol is classed as a reliever and should be used when an asthma attack occurs or prior to engaging in an activity that might make a patient breathless, such as playing sport. Beclometasone is classed as a preventer and, if taken regularly, should improve breathing and reduce the need for the patient to use the salbutamol reliever. The beclometasone will have no impact on relieving an attack when it has already started. Patients who understand the purpose of each of these inhalers are more likely to be able to use them at the appropriate times.

An increasing number of organizations store some or all of their medical records electronically. Storing the records electronically allows them to be searched. Pharmacists searching through a patient's medical notes can help to identify which patients might benefit from a medication review; for example, records can be searched to identify patients with a diagnosis of asthma who might be over-using their reliever inhaler and under-using their preventer inhaler. Pharmacists can also search the electronic records to identify which medicines which might be missing. For example, patients with angina are at greater risk of suffering from a myocardial infarction and should be assessed for an antiplatelet drug; so pharmacists can search through medical notes to identify patients with a diagnosis of angina but who have not been given an antiplatelet medicine such as aspirin.

Patients should be involved in medication reviews. This not only allows the patient to provide information on control of any symptoms they may have but also to take part in any decision-making. Concordance applies to medication reviews just as much as it applies to prescribing medicines. Medication reviews provide patients with an opportunity to find out more about their condition and treatment.

> ### KEY POINT
>
> Reviewing the appropriateness of prescribed medication has the potential to improve health outcomes and improve the efficiency of medication use. Pharmacists have an important role to play and it is important that they prepare beforehand and involve the patient in the review.

> ### SELF CHECK 8.2
>
> You have been asked to review Mahendra Patel's (age 62) regular prescription for naproxen 250 mg tablets. How will you prepare for this review and what questions will you ask?

CASE STUDY 8.2

Reviewing how a patient uses his medicine

Mr PM presents the following prescription to his local community pharmacy:

- Amlodipine 5 mg tablets, one to be taken daily.

- Simvastatin 20 mg tablets, one to be taken daily.

- Bendroflumethiazide 2.5 mg tablets, one to taken daily.

REFLECTION QUESTIONS

1. What legal checks should you undertake?

2. What clinical checks should you undertake?

3. What are the therapeutic outcomes for this patient?

4. How can we monitor the therapeutic outcomes?

5. What are the safety outcomes for this patient? How can we monitor the safety outcomes?

6. What will the cost be?

7. Does the patient have any problems taking the medicines?

Answers

1. Has the prescription been written correctly? Does it contain all the required information such as particulars of the prescriber, and is it signed and dated?
   - Is the prescriber authorized to prescribe these items?
   - Has the patient had these medicines before?
   - It would be wise to review the patient medication record first to see if he is a regular patient.

2. Are the dosages within the usual range specified in the product literature (Summary of Product Characteristics and BNF). Before any final judgement can be made on appropriateness of the dosage regimen we need to know the indications for each of his medicines, which could be found out by discussing with Mr PM.
   - Do any of the drugs that Mr PM is taking interact? The BNF 'Class of interactions' reports that there is an enhanced hypotensive effect when calcium-channel blockers are given with diuretics.

3.
   - *Hypertension:* to reduce blood pressure below target threshold. For a patient with no atherosclerotic disease or other problems the target is 130/90 mmHg.
   - *Lipids:* to reduce the risk of myocardial infarction.

4. Blood pressure and blood lipid measurements are required to monitor the therapeutic outcomes for this patient. Some pharmacists do perform such tests but these are generally carried out within the general practice. The pharmacist could ask the patient when they last had these measured and if it was more than a year previously could recommend that the patient visits their general practice to have these rechecked.

5. To prevent adverse effects. All of these medicines have a long list of side effects and it would not be possible to explore each possible side effect. It would be worth asking the patient if they have experienced any unpleasant effects since they started taking these medicines and in particular ask the patient whether they are suffering postural hypotension. This is likely to manifest as feeling dizzy when rising.

6. Does the patient have to pay for his prescriptions? Are these private or NHS prescriptions? If they are NHS and the prescription was issued in England is the patient exempt from NHS charges?

7. The medicines are all to be taken once per day, but does the patient know what time each medicine should be taken? The diuretic (bendroflumethiazide) should be taken in the morning as it increases urine output; the statin (simvastatin) should be taken in the evening; and the calcium-channel blocker (amlodipine) can be taken any time. The pharmacist should determine if the patient knows why they are taking each of the medications and also explore whether they remember to take the medicines at the appropriate times.

8.4 The future

The relationships between health professionals and patients are likely to evolve over the coming years, changing the role of pharmacists and the services they provide. This section will attempt to describe the possible evolution of pharmaceutical services and consider the likely impact on professionalism.

Treating minor ailments

Pharmacists have a very long tradition in treating minor ailments. The availability of a specialist health care professional who is able to advise patients on minor health care issues is likely to continue to be an important part of the community pharmacist's role. In recent years there has been a trend for medicines that are only available with a prescription to become available from a pharmacy after several years of use have demonstrated the safety profile of the medicine. There is also a trend for pharmacy-only medicines to become available through other retail outlets without input from a pharmacist. The range of medicines that pharmacists have to treat minor ailments is therefore likely to change over time.

Prescribing

The National Insurance Act 1911 drew a distinction between prescribing and dispensing when it made it clear that doctors should prescribe and pharmacists should dispense. This distinction between prescribing and dispensing, which has stood for a century, is becoming blurred as pharmacists take on a prescribing role in addition to dispensing. Pharmacist prescribers must ensure that their principles are not compromised by taking on prescribing and they should clearly separate the prescribing and dispensing roles.

 See Chapter 1 for more on the history of pharmacy.

Pharmacists who have completed the 48-day prescribing course have been able to prescribe medicines since 2006. The proportion of pharmacists who can prescribe is still relatively low but is increasing. These prescribing pharmacists will have much greater control over medicine selection and their expertise on efficacy, safety, cost, and patient

acceptability should have a positive impact on health care outcomes and costs.

Public health

A great many of the health problems that the UK population faces are aggravated by lifestyle factors. The risk of developing cardiovascular disease is raised by smoking, poor diet, and lack of exercise. Type 2 diabetes is associated with obesity.

Screening at-risk patients and intervening with appropriate therapies combined with lifestyle advice and support can have a major impact on public health. Pharmacists can play a major part in screening and treatment programmes to improve health outcomes and this is likely to increase in the future.

Technology has improved over the years such that diagnostic testing does not require a laboratory. Such testing could easily be carried out within pharmacies. Pharmacists have the training to perform such tests and to interpret the results. Communication skills are covered in all schools of pharmacy and these may have to be developed a stage further if pharmacists become involved in providing patients with test results that could be very sensitive.

Personalized medicine

In the future it is likely that personalized medicine will play an increasingly larger part of the pharmacist role. It is known that genetic variations are responsible for differences in rates of metabolism of certain medicines. It is also known that a patient's genetic code can be used to predict the likelihood that certain medicines will have the desired therapeutic effect or harmful effects. Genetic testing of patients to help identify the most suitable doses of a medicine for individual patients, or to match patients to specific medicines, are aspects of personalized medicine.

➤ This chapter described the pharmacist's unique contribution to patient care. It focused on problem-solving to achieve pharmaceutical care.

➤ A medicine's effectiveness, safety, cost, and its acceptability to patients should be considered when comparing treatment options.

➤ When reviewing the evidence regarding benefit or harm associated with a particular medicine it is important to review the quality of the evidence.

➤ Pharmaceutical care involves taking responsibility for setting therapeutic outcomes for an individual patient that will improve their quality of life, and monitoring the effectiveness and safety of the therapy.

FURTHER READING

Drug interactions

Appendix 1 of the *British National Formulary* and *Stockley's Drug Interactions* are the most commonly consulted sources of information on drug interactions. *Stockley's Drug Interactions* provides a far greater amount of detail on the incidence, mechanism, and potential consequences of interactions to support their management. The availability of the *British National Formulary* to pharmacists and pharmacy students means that in practice it is more frequently consulted.

Baxter, K (Ed). *Stockley's Drug Interactions*. 9th edn. Pharmaceutical Press, 2010.

Regulation of medicines and pharmacovigilance

The Medicines and Healthcare products Regulatory Agency (MHRA) has produced a document entitled *Medicines and Medical Devices Regulation: What You Need to Know*. The pdf can be downloaded freely from the MHRA website. It addresses what the MHRA does with respect to its licensing and monitoring roles.

The section at the front of the *British National Formulary* on adverse drug reactions is also useful.

Pharmacoeconomics

An understanding of the economics affecting health care is vital for pharmacists and pharmacy students. The discussion in this chapter is intended as an introduction only. If you require more in-depth coverage of pharmacoeconomics you should consult one of the following texts:

Elliot, R. and Payne, K. *Essentials of Economic Evaluation in Health care*. Pharmaceutical Press, 2005.

National Institute for Health and Clinical Excellence. *Measuring Effectiveness and Cost Effectiveness: The QALY*. <http://www.nice.org.uk/newsroom/features/measuringeffectivenessandcosteffectivenesstheqaly.jsp>.

Glossary

Adherence The extent to which the patient's behaviour matches *agreed* recommendations from the prescriber.

Auscultation Listening to the sounds made by organs such as the heart and lungs.

Balance of probabilities The standard of proof required in civil cases.

Burden of proof The obligation of a party to prove its allegations.

Case law Any set of rulings on law which is guided by previous rulings (also referred to as common law).

Caution Details of any precautions or special monitoring required

Cholera The most dreaded of the infectious disease epidemics of the nineteenth century. Cholera is an infection of the small intestine that causes a large amount of watery diarrhoea. It is caused by the bacterium *Vibrio cholerae* and is transmitted in contaminated food or water. The disease strikes quickly, often killing within hours and leaving the victim a wizened caricature of their former self.

Claimant The party who initiates a civil law suit (formerly referred to as the plaintiff).

Climate change A long-term change in the earth's climate, most commonly associated with change due to an increase in the average atmospheric temperature.

Clinical audit Review of the provision of care against a set of explicit criteria, such as National Institute for Health and Clinical Excellence (NICE) guidance. The clinical audit should specify what standard is expected and this could be that 100% of patients are treated according to the NICE guidance. If the review highlights any areas that fall short of the standards then action should be taken (intervention) to address the issues. This can become a clinical audit cycle with repeated reviewing and interventions.

Clinical governance A framework through which NHS organizations are accountable for continuously improving the quality of their services and safeguarding high standards of care by creating an environment in which excellence in clinical care will flourish. It involves setting standards, monitoring the care provided, and all actions that are taken to ensure that the standards are met.

Clinical management plan (CMP) An agreement drawn up by independent and supplementary prescribers that specifies the types of medicine that can be prescribed, the clinical conditions that can be treated by the supplementary prescriber, and specific indications that should be referred back to the independent prescriber. Each CMP should be produced for a named patient. The CMP is produced on a standard form produced by the Department of Health.

Cognition The mental processes involved in gaining knowledge and comprehension, including processing information from our everyday lives and using our memories of past behaviour to make sense of that information.

Common law Any set of rulings on law which is guided by previous rulings (also referred to as case law).

Comorbidity When a patient has two or more conditions which are unrelated.

Concordance Where the prescriber and patient negotiate as equals to agree a plan of treatment that respects the beliefs and wishes of the patient in determining whether, when, and how medicines are to be taken.

Contraindication Circumstances when a drug should not be used.

Demographics Characteristics of people that characterize them as part of a population. Some of these might be age, sex, race, and level of education. These factors can help us to identify groups within a population that are more likely to do certain things than others and can also be used to explain why people do the things they do.

Devolution The process of diverting power away from centralized government to the regions (most commonly perceived in the UK as the diversion of power away from government at Westminster to governments in Cardiff, Edinburgh, and Belfast).

Epidemiology The scientific study of the distribution of disease and injury.

Evidence-based medicine Systematically finding, appraising, and using research to inform clinical decision-making.

Gross national product (GNP) per capita GNP per capita is the total volume of all final goods and services produced by a country's factors of production and sold on the market in a given time period (usually 1 year) per head of the population.

Holistic Taking all aspects of a patient's well-being into account. It could include considering their physical condition, mental health, social needs, and spiritual health when investigating symptoms and selecting treatment.

Human immunodeficiency virus/acquired immunodeficiency syndrome (HIV/AIDS) HIV is a retrovirus that infects cells of the immune system, destroying or impairing their function. The most advanced stage of HIV infection is acquired immunodeficiency syndrome (AIDS). HIV is transmitted through unprotected sexual intercourse, sharing of contaminated needles, transfusion of contaminated blood, and between a mother and her infant during pregnancy, childbirth, and breastfeeding. The majority of HIV infections are acquired through unprotected sexual intercourse. Such transmission can be effectively prevented by the use of either male or female condoms.

Independent prescriber Takes responsibility for a patient's clinical assessment and diagnosis. In general, takes responsibility for prescribing any medication that the patient may require but may agree to share the responsibility for ongoing prescribing with a supplementary prescriber.

Indication A clinical use for a medicine.

Indictable offence The case is heard at the Crown Court (in relation to the legal system in England and Wales).

Indictment The document containing the charges against the defendant for trial in the Crown Court (in relation to the legal system in England and Wales).

Meta-analysis Statistically combining the results of several clinical trials. It can help to identify trends and patterns because several samples are combined.

Nanny state A negative perception of over-bearing state intervention, such as a government introducing regulations to ensure its population behaves in a certain way.

National Institute for Health and Excellence (NICE) Body that collates and evaluates evidence on health care and shares best practice.

National Patient Safety Agency (NPSA) Body responsible for ensuring that there is a coordinated approach to protecting patient safety and that lessons are learnt from previous incidents and this information is shared to minimize the risk of the same mistake happening again.

Obesity A condition in which excess body fat has accumulated to the degree that it may adversely affect health. Body mass index, a measurement which compares height and weight to give a proxy measure of body fat, defines people as obese when greater than 30 kg/m^2.

Off label Off-label use of a medicine involves using a licensed medicine outwith its licensed uses. This could involve prescribing a medicine for a condition for which it has not been licensed or using it in children when the licence covers its use in adults.

Palpation The use of light pressure from the fingers onto the body surface to investigate a patient's symptoms or condition.

Patent Inventors and designers can protect their invention or design by applying for a patent, which prevents other people profiting from the idea. Pharmaceutical companies apply for a patent to cover a new drug or formulation they have developed. A drug patent normally lasts for 20 years.

Percussion Sounds are generated from a patient by striking the fingers over organs as part of a physical examination. Fingers may be struck over a chest to explore whether the amount of air in the chest is normal.

Pharmacodynamics What a drug does to the body. It covers the action of the drug.

Pharmacokinetics What the body does to the drug. It describes how a drug passes through the body (absorption, distribution, metabolism, and excretion).

Pharmacovigilance Pharmacovigilance is the term used to describe the ongoing monitoring of a medicine's safety, the assessment of risk, and informing health professionals and patients regarding a medicines safety.

Phlebotomists Assistant health care scientists who specialize in taking blood samples. Other health care professionals, including pharmacists, can complete phlebotomy training and incorporate this into their standard roles.

Practice nurse A nurses employed by a GP practice whose role is to support the GP in the provision of general medical services such as immunization, health screening, and specialist clinics such as for asthma and diabetes.

Problem-based learning A student-centred style of learning that involves small groups of students working together and directing their own learning to seek solutions to clinical problems. It encourages collaborative working and the development of problem-solving skills.

Protected title A number of job titles, such as architect, doctor, dentist, and pharmacist, are protected by law such that it is an offence for anyone who is not registered with the relevant body to use such a title.

Public interest There is a public interest in good decision-making by public bodies (including the courts) in upholding standards of integrity, in ensuring justice and fair treatment for all, in securing the best use of public resources, and in ensuring fair commercial competition in a mixed economy.

Quality-adjusted life year (QALY) One QALY is equal to 1 year in 'perfect health' for one patient. The QALY can be used to compare the cost benefit of different medical treatments where typically the number of additional QALYs per treatment can be compared for a range of treatments.

Research method The way research is carried out. The way a research question is asked will determine the method used.

Role extension The extension of the pharmacist's role from its traditional functions of drug procurement, compounding, and dispensing to include involvement in direct patient care, clinical services, and public health.

Scottish Intercollegiate Guidelines Network (SIGN) Body that collates and evaluates evidence on health care and shares best practice.

Side effects Effects which are secondary to the main desired effect of a drug. Side effects may be beneficial or harmful.

Socialist An advocate of socialism. Socialism is a theory of social organization that advocates placing the ownership and control of land, capital, and the means of production (factories, mines etc.) in the community as a whole.

Standard of proof The level of proof demanded or required in a specific case, established by assessing the associated evidence. In civil proceedings it is 'on the balance of probabilities'.

Standard operating procedure (SOP) Structured instructions stating what is to be done and by whom. The SOP must specify the activities covered, the objective of the SOP, who is responsible, what the procedure is and describe how the procedure will be audited.

Statute law A system of laws that have been decided and approved by a parliament (or equivalent institution).

Summary offence The case can only be heard in the magistrates' court (in relation to the legal system in England and Wales).

Supplementary prescriber Supplementary prescribing is a voluntary partnership between an independent and a supplementary prescriber that has the agreement of the patient. Supplementary prescribers may take responsibility for prescribing after diagnosis and after a patient-specific clinical management plan (CMP) has been prepared. Supplementary prescribers are permitted to prescribe any medication provided it has been listed in the CMP. The supplementary prescriber can be a nurse, pharmacist, chiropodist, physiotherapist, or optometrist.

Sustainable development A pattern of development which ensures that all people throughout the world are able to satisfy their basic needs while making sure that future generations can enjoy the same quality of life.

Systematic review Reviewing the literature to identify all studies which are relevant to the research question. The process involves assessing the quality of the evidence in the literature and includes only those studies that meet the criteria set by those conducting the review.

Therapeutic drug monitoring (TDM) The use of actual drug levels and the application of pharmacokinetic principles in the clinical situation to individualize drug treatment and to improve patient care.

Triable either way The case can be heard either at the magistrates' court or the Crown Court (in relation to the legal system in England and Wales) and depends on a number of factors, such as the seriousness of the offence(s).

Welfare state The welfare state in the UK was a commitment by the government to provide for people from 'cradle to grave' in matters of health care, education, employment, and social security. Its roots were in the Beveridge Report of 1942, which identified the five 'giant evils' affecting society: squalor, ignorance, want, idleness, and disease. Clement Atlee's 1945 Labour government pledged to eradicate these evils and introduced policies to meet those aims.

White Paper A government report considered to be a statement of policy. It often outlines proposals for legislative change or the introduction of new laws.

Unlicensed A medicine which has not been granted a product licence for use in the European Economic Area (EEA).

Answers to self check questions

Chapter 1

1.1

- Communication skills are vitally important for pharmacists. Pharmacists must be able to ascertain what problems and symptoms the patient has and then be able to discuss options with patients and other health care professionals.

- Mathematical and arithmetical skills are key skills. Understanding and applying research data to patients frequently requires the ability to perform mathematical operations. Dosage calculations require the use of arithmetical skills.

- Practical skills are required when preparing medicines. The extent of extemporaneous preparation of medicines may be lower now than previously, but accurate preparation of medicines is still required when dispensing medicines such as antibiotic suspensions. The practical skills are not only limited to measuring but also include techniques to minimize contamination during aseptic preparation.

1.2

- To compare the occupations it is necessary to review each of the four attributes:

  - *Knowledge*: Pharmacists have access to specialized knowledge which requires a level of understanding sufficient to realize the significance and application of that knowledge. Some high-street retailers may also require specialized knowledge.

  - *Autonomy*: Community pharmacists do not require their work to be checked by any other professional. Other high-street retailers also do not require their work to be checked by another professional, although the work they are engaged in may not be subject to the same level of legal control as that involved in the sale and supply of medicines.

  - *Service orientation*: Pharmacists are bound by a code of ethics, the *Standards for Conduct, Ethics and Performance*. If pharmacists are found to have fallen short of these standards then they can have their name removed from the register of pharmacists. Other high-street retailers do not necessarily have a formal code of ethics by which they have to abide.

  - *Monopoly*: Pharmacist is a restricted title and only those registered with the General Pharmaceutical Council (GPhC) can call themselves a pharmacist. Community pharmacy premises must also be registered with the GPhC. Community pharmacies which dispense NHS prescriptions must have a contract with the NHS to provide pharmaceutical services and there are a number of tests which must be fulfilled prior to obtaining a contract. Most other high-street retailers do not possess a restricted title and do not require registration or a contract before they can trade.

- The four attributes of professionalism can be applied to community pharmacists. Some of the attributes can be applied to some high-street retailers but it is necessary to apply all four for professional status. Many optometrists also occupy a high-street location and the four attributes can be applied to them, indicating their professional status.

1.3
Professionalism

The attributes of professionalism were introduced in Chapter 1. The following question was posed: Is pharmacy a profession? Obviously, it is up to individual readers to answer that question for themselves, but the likely impact on professionalism is considered under each professional attribute described in Chapter 1.

- *Knowledge*: The gap in knowledge between professionals and patients is likely to reduce, at least for some patients. It is, however, hard to envisage a time when this gap will have completely disappeared. Pharmacists should welcome the reduction in the knowledge gap because it will allow them to provide a greater depth of information to those patients who are better informed.

- *Monopoly*: There is continual change in the range of medicines which are available to purchase from retail outlets and pharmacies. As a medicine becomes more established and its safety profile better understood it is more likely to be reclassified as a medicine which can be sold from a pharmacy (class P medicine) or a medicine which can be sold from other retail outlets (general sale list medicine). There are many medicines which can now be purchased from supermarkets that 20 years ago were only available on a prescription from a doctor. It is likely that this trend will continue. Pharmacies may lose their monopoly over certain medicines but at the same time it is likely that they will be able to sell other medicines that previously could only be supplied via a prescription.

- *Autonomy*: A number of high-profile cases involving poor practice by medical practitioners led to the introduction of lay members to the ruling council of the health profession regulators. It is unlikely the balance will move further towards the lay public but that is largely dependent upon public confidence in the ability of the health profession regulators to regulate their professions and the manner in which they deal with poorly performing members of their profession.

- *Service orientation*: A relatively small but nevertheless increasing proportion of a pharmacy's income is derived from the delivery of services for which they are paid a flat fee, in a similar manner to other professions.

1.4 Students will come into contact with patients and the public during their training. Ensuring students are fit to practise will help to:

- Ensure the safety of patients and the public.
- Maintain the public's confidence in the profession.

Chapter 2

2.1 New drug treatments are available for previously unmanaged or poorly controlled conditions and demand for medical intervention to meet health needs has increased.

2.2 Health care professionals who have a contract with the NHS and are not directly employed by the NHS.

2.3 GPs know their patients better than managers and can balance an individual patient's needs against other patients' medical needs.

2.4 It allows pharmacists to demonstrate that they are providing high-quality services to their patients.

Chapter 3

3.1
   a. High Court case: Mr Roderick. Court of Appeal case: Mrs Dwyer. In case law, the name of the claimant appears first and after the 'v' one finds the name(s) of the defendant(s).

   b. On the balance of probabilities.

   c. The burden of proof lies with the claimant (plaintiff).

3.2 Defamation is an example of a civil case where trial by jury can be requested.

3.3 The four main principles in health care ethics are autonomy (respecting the choice/decision of an individual), non-maleficence (avoiding harm), beneficence (promoting well-being or doing good), and justice (similar individuals should normally have access to the same health care, together with consideration of the fair distribution of limited resources).

3.4 A class P medicine can be lawfully supplied to a member of the public without a prescription from a registered pharmacy by a pharmacist or by someone under the supervision of a pharmacist.

3.5 14 years.

3.6 A pharmacist may lawfully possess drugs in Schedule 2, 3, 4-1, 4-2, and 5 (all except Schedule 1) without the need of a licence from the Home Office.

3.7 Only the Fitness to Practise Committee has the power to remove a pharmacist's name from the register.

3.8
   a. High Court
   b. Court of Session

Chapter 4

4.1 Upstream factors include social, physical, economic, and environmental factors. Downstream factors include individual lifestyle factors (such as smoking, alcohol intake, and diet) and demographic and hereditary factors over which an individual has no influence.

4.2 The public health approach highlights the collective responsibility for improvement in health and prevention of disease. Anybody with an ability to influence health should use it to improve the health of the population. This includes teachers, transport engineers, social workers, health visitors, environmental health officers, pharmacists, nurses, dentists, and doctors.

4.3 The main causes of the outbreaks were poor housing, overcrowding, and insanitary conditions (limited access to clean drinking water and no sewerage systems).

4.4 The creation of the NHS meant that for the first time, workers' dependents, the poor, and those requiring specialist services were able to access suitable health care.

4.5 The idea that individuals can be 'nudged' (for example, by increasing the prominence of healthy food in eateries) to adopt a healthier lifestyle rather than the government having to intervene to influence behavioural change (by, for example, banning unhealthy practices).

4.6 The creation of the NHS led to a steep increase in the volume of state prescriptions. To meet this increased workload pharmacists relocated from 'front of house' to dispensary.

4.7 The three levels of the contract are essential, advanced, and enhanced. Public health is described as an essential service obliging all pharmacy contractors to provide it. Numerous 'pharmacy public health' interventions are included in the enhanced level.

4.8 In low-income countries, communicable (infectious) disease is the primary cause of death and disease. In high-income countries, non-communicable (chronic) diseases such as cancers and cardiovascular disease are the primary cause of death and disease.

4.9 The current public health practice of community pharmacists is focused on downstream interventions such as health promotion. Pharmacists tend to focus on individual behaviour (that is, lifestyles) rather than the wider determinants of health that are the focus of the wider public health movement.

Chapter 5

5.1 Venlafaxine is an antidepressant. Diclofenac is a non-steroidal anti-inflammatory drug.

- Is it a new therapy?
  - Yes, the diclofenac is new.
- Is the medication indicated?
  - We do not know the exact nature of James's injury but diclofenac is indicated for soft tissue injuries. We could explore with James how he hurt his leg.
- Is it appropriate and recommended (evidence-based medicine or local guidelines)?
  - The *BNF* recommends analgesics as first-line treatment for soft tissue injuries. We don't know whether James has tried taking paracetamol so we could explore this with him.

- Is the formulation appropriate?
  - It is available as a topical preparation but this is generally more expensive. The *BNF* suggests considering this. The efficacy is similar but the adverse event profile is likely to be different. James can take tablets (as he is already taking venlafaxine).
- Are there any cautions?
  - There are a range of cautions such as use in the elderly or concurrent diuretics, but these do not apply in this case.
- Are there any contraindications?
  - Previous or current peptic ulcer is a contraindication. We should ask James whether he has had any previous gastric problems.
- Is the dose appropriate?
  - Yes.
- Are there any interactions (existing drug or disease)?
  - Yes, there is an increased risk of bleeding when taking diclofenac with venlafaxine.
- Is the patient allergic?
  - We have no information. We should ask whether James has taken this previously and if he suffered any problems while taking it.
- Is the duration appropriate?
  - Yes.

This prescription is not appropriate for James owing to the interaction with venlafaxine. It would be worth speaking to James to determine what action he has tried so far before speaking to the prescriber. Depending upon the responses that James provides it may be worth recommending paracetamol.

5.2 See Appendix 3 of the *BNF* for the labels.

a. Fifty-six propranolol 80 MR capsules for Rachel Vickers, aged 31:
- Label 8
- Label 25

b. Azithromycin capsules for Dilip Patel, aged 55:
- Label 5
- Label 9
- Label 23

c. Fourteen doxycycline 100 mg capsules for Ravi Patel:
- Label 6
- Label 9
- Label 11
- Label 27
- Counselling posture: capsules should be taken whole with plenty of fluid during meals while standing or sitting.

d. 100 ml chlorphenamine syrup for Maya Vickers, aged 3:
- Label 2 but probably not necessary to include the last part of the warning about avoiding alcohol.

Chapter 6

6.1 In the current health care system, patients are increasingly cared for by multidisciplinary teams involving a wide range of health care and other professionals.

6.2 In 2000 in London 8-year-old Victoria Climbié, from the Ivory Coast, was tortured and murdered by her guardians, one of whom was her great-aunt. Her death led to a public inquiry and produced major changes in child protection policies in England, including the 'Every Child Matters' initiative.

6.3 These could be any of the health and social care professionals listed in this chapter.

6.4 Interprofessional education is an interactive development of the more didactic shared learning and has been defined as: 'Occasions when two or more professions learn with, from and about each other to improve collaboration and the quality of care.' (Centre for the Advancement of Interprofessional Education, 2002).

6.5 Problem-based learning is when students are given a problem based on a real-life situation or scenario. Each scenario is carefully designed by experts to expose students to the information and skills that they need. These scenarios can be for individuals or groups.

6.6

1. Preparing the environment: establishing initial rapport with the patient and identifying the reason(s) for the consultation.

2. Exploring the problem by gathering information from the practitioner and the patient perspective to set it in context.

3. Building the relationship and establishing patient involvement.

4. Providing structure and signposting to the interview.

5. Explaining the process and achieving a shared understanding.

6. Closing the interview and developing a forward plan.

Chapter 7

7.1

- Intention does not always result in actual behaviour. We can say we intend to do something over and over again but not necessarily do it.
- The model does not take into account people's beliefs about the amount of control they have over the behaviour in question.
- The model does not address the order of beliefs or direction of causality.

But

- The theory of planned behaviour (TPB) has been widely tested and successfully applied.
- It incorporates important cognitive variables.
- It acknowledges that the role of social pressure is important.
- TPB includes role of past behaviour.

7.2

- They might come into the pharmacy and ask for help or they might come in and ask about whether there is anything they can buy that will help them lose weight. This would give you the opportunity to ask whether they were thinking of going on a diet.

- If they said they were thinking of going on a diet you might first want to check whether they have dieted before and whether this was successful. This would give you a clue as to what type of support you could offer. If they had any health problems (such as diabetes) you should suggest that they check with their doctor first, before starting a diet.

- You could advise them on what to eat so that they would not feel hungry, how often to weigh themselves, and could offer them the opportunity of coming into your pharmacy to be weighed regularly. This would give you a chance to keep them motivated by encouraging them to stick with the diet.

- You could suggest they keep a food diary so that they can see what they are eating each day.

- Remember—failure is OK. The important thing is that you keep in contact with people so that you are there to offer help in the future.

7.3 Once a person has started a diet the most important thing for them is to see their weight begin to reduce. At this stage you could encourage them to stick to their diet and give them lots of praise when that first kilo disappears. You can also keep them going when they do not lose weight by encouraging them to see that they have already lost 1 kilo and so they can do it! You could also:

- agree with them a date for starting the diet;

- go through their diary with them to suggest how they could make changes and you could propose healthy, nutritious alternatives;

- help them decide how much weight they want to lose and agree a target date;

- make an appointment for them to come and see you each week to be weighed.

7.4 This sort of question is the reason why you need to understand how to interpret health research. To answer a prescriber who asks about the safety of two different medicines you would need to have read the research data about both medicines and be able to tell the prescriber your decision, using that information to back you up. What is most important about giving advice about medicines is to be able to say you do not know (if that is the case) but that you do know where to source the information and can find the answer.

Chapter 8

8.1

Naina Patel, aged 54. Diagnosed 3 years ago with type 2 diabetes mellitus. She is currently prescribed metformin 500 mg.

- Maintain blood glucose concentration between 4 and 9 mmol/litre.

Suresh Shah, aged 52. Diagnosed with angina 5 years ago. He is currently prescribed atenolol 50 mg and glyceryl trinitrate 500 µg.

- Prevent anginal attacks from occurring.

- Treat anginal attacks when do occur.

- Prevent myocardial infarction.

8.2

- You will need to know the indication for Mahendra's medicine. Naproxen is used for rheumatoid arthritis (RA), gout, and other musculoskeletal problems. You could contact the surgery or you could ask Mahendra when he arrives for the review.

- You could check your patient medication records to see how long he has been talking naproxen, how frequently he collects it, and whether anything else has been tried in the past. It is worth noting that Mahendra may have visited other community pharmacies so your records may not have all the information.

- Does Mahendra know why he is taking the medication?
  - If for RA or another musculoskeletal problem then you could ask how well it is controlling the pain and inflammation. You could ask if he has tried anything else prior to taking the naproxen.
  - If for gout you should ask how frequently he has attacks of gout and how well the naproxen deals with the attacks. If attacks are frequent then a prophylactic drug may be of use (see *BNF* 10.1.4).

- Does he use it as prescribed?

- Does he have any problems ordering, obtaining, taking, or using the medicine?

- You should explore with Mahendra how long he has been taking the naproxen and whether he suffers any discomfort while taking it. These drugs are cautioned in elderly patients so particular attention should be paid to possible adverse effects (see *BNF* 10.1).

- Could formulations/dosages be optimized to improve adherence or improve cost effectiveness? You should review different formulations of naproxen listed in the *BNF*.

Bibliography

Chapter 1

Anderson, S. *Making Medicines: A Brief History of Pharmacy and Pharmaceuticals*. Pharmaceutical Press, 2005.

Copeman, W.S.C. *Apothecaries of London: A History 1617–1967*. Pergamon Press, 1967.

David, T.J., Schafheutle, E.I., and Hall, J. Fitness-to-practise procedures for pharmacy students and how they work. *Pharmaceutical Journal* 2009; 282: 646–7.

David, T., Schafheutle, E.I., and Hall, J. What 'fitness to practise' means for school and students' behaviour. *Pharmaceutical Journal* 2009; 282: 623–4.

Dingwall, H.M. *Physicians, Surgeons and Apothecaries: Medicine in Seventeenth-Century Edinburgh*. Tuckwell Press, 1995.

Earles, M.P. A History of the Society. *Pharmaceutical Journal* 1991; Anniversary Supplement: S6–9.

General Pharmaceutical Council. *Code of Conduct for Pharmacy Students*. GPhC, 2010. <http://www.msp.ac.uk/documents/gphcstudentscodeofconductv02_small.pdf> [Accessed 17 Jan 2013].

General Pharmaceutical Council. *Criteria for Initial Registration as a Pharmacy Technician*. GPhC, 2011. <http://www.pharmacyregulation.org/sites/default/files/Criteria%20for%20initial%20registration%20as%20a%20pharmacy%20technician%20Oct%202011.pdf> [Accessed 17 January 2013].

General Pharmaceutical Council. *Future Pharmacists: Standards for the Initial Education and Training of Pharmacists*. GPhC, 2011. <http://www.pharmacyregulation.org/sites/default/files/Standards%20for%20the%20initial%20education%20and%20training%20of%20pharmacists.pdf> [Accessed 17 January 2013].

General Pharmaceutical Council. *Guidance on Student Fitness to Practise Procedures in Schools of Pharmacy*. GPhC, 2010. <http://www.pharmacyregulation.org> [Accessed 17 January 2013].

General Pharmaceutical Council. *Pharmacist Independent Prescribing Programme: Learning Outcomes and Indicative Content*. GPhC, 2012 <http://www.pharmacyregulation.org/sites/default/files/Pharmacist%20Independent%20Prescribing%20-%20Learning%20Outcomes%20and%20Indicative%20Content.pdf> [Accessed 17 January 2013].

General Pharmaceutical Council. *Raising concerns*. <http://www.pharmacyregulation.org/raising-concerns> [Accessed 17 January 2013].

General Pharmaceutical Council. *Standards for Conduct, Ethics and Performance*. GPhC, 2010. <http://www.pharmacyregulation.org/sites/default/files/Standards%20of%20conduct,%20ethics%20and%20performance.pdf>.

Hall, J., David, T., and Tully, M. *Fitness to Practise Issues and Ethical Dilemmas Encountered by Pharmacy Students and Pre-Registration Trainees*. University of Manchester, 2011. <http://www.pharmacyregulation.org/sites/default/files/Fitness%20to%20practise%20issues.pdf> [Accessed 17 January 2013].

Holloway, S.W.F. *Royal Pharmaceutical Society of Great Britain 1841–1991: A Political and Social History*. Pharmaceutical Press, 1991.

Mathews, L.G. *History of Pharmacy in Britain*. W & S Livingstone, 1962.

Medicines and Healthcare products Regulatory Agency. *Medicines and Medical Devices Regulation: What You Need to Know*. MHRA, 2008. <http://www.mhra.gov.uk/home/groups/comms-ic/documents/websiteresources/con2031677.pdf> [Accessed 17 January 2013].

Office for National Statistics. Standard Occupational Classification 2010. ONS, 2010. <http://www.ons.gov.uk/ons/guide-method/classifications/current-standard-classifications/soc2010/soc2010-volume-1-structure-and-descriptions-of-unit-groups/index.html> [Accessed 17 January 2013].

Parmar, H. and Hall, J. Behaviour is assessed before a would-be students starts a university course. *Pharmaceutical Journal* 2010; 285: 123–4.

Parsons, T. *The Social System*. Routledge and Kegan Paul, 1951.

Royal Pharmaceutical Society. *Medicines Ethics and Practice: The Professional Guide for Pharmacists*. Pharmaceutical Press, 2011.

Scambler, G. *Sociology as Applied to Medicine*. 5th edn. Saunders, 2003.

Society of Apothecaries. <http://www.apothecaries.org/society/our-history/>.

Chapter 2

Scotland

The Scottish Government. *NHS workforce*. <http://www.scotland.gov.uk/Topics/Health/NHS-Scotland> [Accessed 17 January 2013].

Northern Ireland

Department of Health, Social Services and Public Safety. *About the department*. <http://www.dhsspsni.gov.uk/index/about_dept.htm> [Accessed 17 January 2013].

Wales

NHS Wales. *Health in Wales*. <http://www.wales.nhs.uk> [Accessed 17 January 2013].

England

Department of Health. *Public health, adult social care, and the NHS.* <http://www.dh.gov.uk> [Accessed 17 January 2013].

Chapter 3

Appelbe, G.E. and Wingfield, J. (Eds). Dale and Appelbe's Pharmacy Law and Ethics. 9th edn. Pharmaceutical Press, 2009.

Electronic Medicines Compendium. <http://www.medicines.org.uk/emc> [Accessed 7 May 2012].

General Pharmaceutical Council. <http://www.pharmacyregulation.org> [Accessed 7 May 2012].

General Pharmaceutical Council. Fitness to practise committee. <http://www.pharmacyregulation.org/raising-concerns/hearings/committees/fitness-practise-committee> [Accessed 7 May 2012].

Home Office. Drugs and the law. <http://www.homeoffice.gov.uk/drugs/drug-law> [Accessed 7 May 2012].

Medicines and Healthcare products Regulatory Agency. <http://www.mhra.gov.uk> [Accessed 7 May 2012].

Mullan, K. Writing a wrong. *British Medical Journal* 1988; 297: 470.

Pharmaceutical Society of Northern Ireland. <http://www.psni.org.uk> [Accessed 7 May 2012].

Professional Standards Authority for Health and Social Care (formerly Council for Healthcare Regulatory Excellence). <http://www.chre.org.uk> [Accessed 7 May 2012].

Veterinary Medicines Directorate. <http://www.vmd.defra.gov.uk> [Accessed 7 May 2012].

Chapter 4

Public Health: A Practical Guide for Community Pharmacists. Pharmaceutical Services Negotiating Committee, National Pharmaceutical Association, Royal Pharmaceutical Society of Great Britain, and PharmacyHealthLink, 2004. <http://www.npa.co.uk/Documents/Docstore/PCO_LPCs/Public_Health.pdf>.

What future for general practice pharmacists? *Pharmaceutical Journal* 1981; 227: 300–1.

Acheson, D. *Public Health in England: Report of the Committee of the Inquiry into the Future Development of the Public Health Function.* Department of Health, 1988.

Anderson, S. The changing role of the community pharmacist in health promotion in Great Britain 1930 to 1995. *Pharmaceutical Historian* 2002; 32: 7–10.

Baggott, R. *Public Health: Policy and Politics.* Palgrave, 2000.

Bevan, A. *In place of fear.* New edn. Wakefield: EP Publishing, 1976.

Beveridge, W. *Social Insurance and Allied Services.* HMSO, 1942.

Birenbaum, A. Reprofessionalization in pharmacy. *Social Science and Medicine* 1982; 16: 871–8.

Birmingham City Council. Historic population of Birmingham. <http://www.birmingham.gov.uk/cs/Satellite?c=Page&childpagename=Lib-Central-Archives-and-Heritage%2FPageLayout&cid=1223092760414&pagename=BCC%2FCommon%2FWrapper%2FWrapper> [Accessed: 22 August 2011].

Bissell, P. and Traulsen, J. M. *Sociology and Pharmacy Practice.* Pharmaceutical Press, 2005.

Black, D. The Black Report. In P. Townsend and N. Davidson (Eds.) *Inequalities in Health.* Penguin, 1988.

Campbell, E., Scadding, J., and Roberts, R. The concept of disease. *British Medical Journal* 1979; ii: 757–62.

Chadwick, E. *Report on the Sanitary Condition of the Labouring Population of Great Britain 1842.* Edinburgh University Press, 1965.

Community Pharmacy Scotland. *NHS care services.* <http://www.communitypharmacyscotland.org.uk/nhs_care_services/nhs_care_services.asp> [Accessed 22 August 2011].

Conisbee, M. *Ghost Town Britain: A Lethal Prescription. The Impact of Deregulation on Community Pharmacies.* New Economics Foundation, 2003.

Dahlgren, G. and Whitehead, M. *Policies and Strategies to Promote Social Equity in Health.* Stockholm: Institute for Futures Studies, 1991.

Department of Health. *A Vision for Pharmacy in the New NHS.* DoH, 2003. <http://www.dh.gov.uk/prod_consum_dh/groups/dh_digitalassets/@dh/@en/documents/digitalasset/dh_4070099.pdf>.

Department of Health. *Choosing Health: Making Healthy Choices Easier.* DoH, 2004. <http://webarchive.nationalarchives.gov.uk/+/dh.gov.uk/en/publicationsandstatistics/publications/publicationspolicyandguidance/dh_4094550>.

Department of Health. *Choosing Health Through Pharmacy: A Programme for Pharmaceutical Public Health 2005–2015.* DoH, 2005. <http://www.dh.gov.uk/prod_consum_dh/groups/dh_digitalassets/@dh/@en/documents/digitalasset/dh_4107496.pdf>.

Department of Health. *Equity and Excellence: Liberating the NHS.* The Stationery Office, 2010. <http://www.dh.gov.uk/prod_consum_dh/groups/dh_digitalassets/@dh/@en/@ps/documents/digitalasset/dh_117794.pdf>.

Department of Health. *Getting Ahead of the Curve: A Strategy for Combating Infectious Diseases.* DoH, 2002. <http://www.dh.gov.uk/prod_consum_dh/groups/dh_digitalassets/@dh/@en/documents/digitalasset/dh_4060875.pdf>.

Department of Health. *Health of the Nation: A Strategy for Health in England.* HMSO, 1992.

Department of Health. *Healthy Lives, Healthy People: Our Strategy for Public Health in England.* The Stationery Office, 2010. <http://www.dh.gov.uk/prod_consum_dh/groups/dh_digitalassets/documents/digitalasset/dh_127424.pdf>.

Department of Health. *Pharmacy in England: Building on Strengths—Delivering the Future*. DoH, 2008. <http://www.official-documents.gov.uk/document/cm73/7341/7341.pdf>.

Department of Health. *Pharmacy in the Future: Implementing the NHS Plan*. DoH, 2000. <http://www.dh.gov.uk/prod_consum_dh/groups/dh_digitalassets/@dh/@en/documents/digitalasset/dh_4068204.pdf>.

Department of Health. *Saving Lives: Our Healthier Nation*. DoH, 1999. <http://www.archive.official-documents.co.uk/document/cm43/4386/4386.htm>.

Department of Health, Social Services and Public Safety. *Investing for Health*. DHSSPS, 2002.

Department of Health, Social Services and Public Safety. *Making it Better: A Strategy for Pharmacy in the Community*. DHSSPS, 2003. <http://www.dhsspsni.gov.uk/makingitbetter.pdf>.

Eaton, G. and Webb, B. Boundary encroachment: Pharmacists in the clinical setting. *Sociology of Health and Illness* 1979; 1: 69–89.

Faculty of Public Health. What is public health? <http://www.fph.org.uk/what_is_public_health> [Accessed 27 August 2011].

Foresight. *Tackling Obesities: Future Choices. Project Report*. Department for Business, Innovation and Skills, 2007. <http://www.bis.gov.uk/assets/bispartners/foresight/docs/obesity/17.pdf>.

Gilbert, L. Pharmacy's attempts to extend its roles: A case study in South Africa. *Social Science and Medicine* 1998; 47: 153–64.

Hancock, T. Lalonde and beyond: Looking back at 'A New Perspective on the Health of Canadians'. *Health Promotion* 1986; 1: 93–100.

Health Protection Agency. H1N1 (2009) pandemic archive. <http://www.hpa.org.uk/Topics/InfectiousDiseases/InfectionsAZ/PandemicInfluenza/H1N1PandemicArchive> [Accessed 22 August 2011].

Hicks, J. and Allen, G. *A Century of Change: Trends in UK Statistics Since 1900*. House of Commons Library, 1999.

Holloway, S.W., Jewson, N.D., and Mason, D.J. 'Reprofessionalization' or 'occupational imperialism'? Some reflections on pharmacy in Britain. *Social Science and Medicine* 1986; 23: 323–32.

Horgan, J.M.P., Blenkinsopp, A., and McManus, R.J. Evaluation of a cardiovascular disease opportunistic risk assessment pilot ('Heart MOT' service) in community pharmacies. *Journal of Public Health* 2010; 32: 110–16.

Hunter, D.J. *Public Health Policy*. Polity, 2003.

Jesson, J. and Bissell, P. Public health and pharmacy: A critical review. *Critical Public Health* 2006; 16:159–69.

Lalonde, M. *A New Perspective on the Health of Canadians*. Ottawa: Ministry of National Health and Welfare, 1974.

Last, J. (Ed). *Dictionary of Epidemiology*. 2nd edn. Oxford University Press, 1988.

McKeown, T. *The Role of Medicine*. 2nd edn. Basil Blackwell, 1979.

NHS Information Centre. *Statistics on Obesity, Physical Activity and Diet: England, February 2009*. The Health and Social Care Information Centre, 2009. <http://www.ic.nhs.uk/webfiles/publications/opan09/OPAD_Feb_2009_final_revised_Aug11.pdf>.

NHS Scotland. *Partnership for Care*. Scottish Executive, 2003. <http://www.scotland.gov.uk/Publications/2003/02/16476/18730>.

NHS Wales. *Improving Health in Wales: The Future of Primary Care*. National Assembly for Wales, 2001. <http://www.wales.nhs.uk/publications/primcare_e.pdf>.

NHS Wales. *Remedies for Success: A Strategy for Pharmacy in Wales*. Welsh Assembly Government, 2002. <http://www.wales.nhs.uk/documents/PharmacyStrategy.pdf>.

Office for National Statistics. *Statistical Bulletin: Life Expectancy at Birth and at Age 65 for Health Areas in the United Kingdom, 2003–05 to 2007–09*. ONS, 2011. <http://www.ons.gov.uk/ons/rel/subnational-health4/life-expectancy-at-birth-and-at-age-65-for-health-areas-in-the-united-kingdom/2003-05-to-2007-09/statistical-bulletin.pdf>.

Office for National Statistics. *The National Statistics Socio-economic Classification (NS-SEC)*. <http://www.ons.gov.uk/ons/guide-method/classifications/archived-standard-classifications/ns-sec/index.html> [Accessed 27 September 2011].

Peterson, A. and Lupton, D. *The New Public Health; Health and Self in the Age of Risk*. Sage, 1996.

Pharmaceutical Services Negotiating Committee. *The pharmacy contract*. <http://www.psnc.org.uk/pages/introduction.html> [Accessed 22 August 2011].

Pharmaceutical Services Negotiating Committee. *Twenty Healthy Living Pharmacy pathfinder sites announced*. <http://www.psnc.org.uk/news.php/1104/twenty_healthy_living_pharmacy_pathfinder_sites_announced> [Accessed 22 August 2011].

Public Health Institute for Scotland. *Pharmacy for Health: The Way Forward for Pharmaceutical Public Health in Scotland*. NHS Scotland, 2002. <http://www.healthscotland.com/uploads/documents/pharmacy.pdf>.

Scottish Executive. *The Right Medicine: A Strategy for Pharmaceutical Care in Scotland*. Scottish Executive, 2002. <http://www.scotland.gov.uk/Resource/Doc/158742/0043086.pdf>.

Snow, J. *On the Mode of Communication of Cholera*. John Churchill, 1855.

Soanes, C. and Stevenson, A. (Eds). *The Concise Oxford English Dictionary*. 12th edn. Oxford University Press, 2008.

Thaler, R. and Sunstein, C. *Nudge: Improving Decisions about Health, Wealth, and Happiness*. New Haven, CT: Yale University Press, 2008.

The Nuffield Foundation. *Pharmacy: The Report of a Committee of Inquiry Appointed by the Nuffield Foundation*. The Nuffield Foundation, 1986.

The Times. 1 August 1854.

Turner, P. The Nuffield report: A signpost for pharmacy. *British Medical Journal* 1986; 292: 1031–3.

United Nations. UNdata, 2011. <http://data.un.org/> [Accessed 22 August 2011].

UNAIDS and World Health Organization. *AIDS Epidemic Update*. WHO, 2009. <http://www.unaids.org/en/media/ unaids/contentassets/dataimport/pub/report/2009/ jc1700_epi_update_2009_en.pdf>.

UNICEF and World Health Organization. *Diarrhoea: Why Children Are Still Dying and What Can Be Done.* WHO, 2009. <http://www.unicef.org/health/files/Final_ Diarrhoea_Report_October_2009_final.pdf>.

Wanless, D. *Securing Good Health for the Whole Population*. Final Report. HM Treasury, 2004. <http://www. dh.gov.uk/en/Publicationsandstatistics/Publications/ PublicationsPolicyAndGuidance/DH_4074426>.

Wanless, D. *Securing Our Future Health: Taking a Long-Term View*. Final Report. HM Treasury, 2002. <http:// webarchive.nationalarchives.gov.uk/+/http:/www. hm-treasury.gov.uk/consult_wanless_final.htm>.

Wilkinson, R. *Unhealthy Societies: The Afflictions of Inequality*. Routledge, 1996.

Wilkinson, R. and Pickett, K. *The Spirit Level: Why More Equal Societies Almost Always Do Better*. Allen Lane, 2009.

World Health Organization. *Constitution of the World Health Organization*. 45th edn. WHO, 2006. <http://www. who.int/governance/eb/who_constitution_en.pdf>.

World Health Organization. *Evolution of a pandemic: A(H1N1) 2009. April 2009—March 2010*. WHO, 2010. <http://whqlibdoc.who.int/publications/2010/ 9789241599924_eng.pdf>.

World Health Organization. *Global Health Observatory Data Repository, 2011: Mortality and Burden of Disease.* <http://apps.who.int/gho/data/> [Accessed 22 August 2011].

World Health Organization. *Protecting Health From Climate Change: Connecting Science, Policy and People*. WHO, 2009. <http://whqlibdoc.who.int/ publications/2009/9789241598880_eng.pdf>.

World Health Organization. *The World Health Report: Working Together for Health*. WHO, 2006. <http://www. who.int/entity/whr/2006/whr06_en.pdf>.

World Health Organization. *Water, Sanitation and Hygiene Links to Health: Facts and Figures Updated March 2004*. WHO, 2004. <http://www.who.int/water_ sanitation_health/publications/facts2004/en/> [Accessed 22 August 2011].

World Health Organization. *World Malaria Report 2010*. WHO, 2010. <http://www.who.int/entity/malaria/world_ malaria_report_2010/worldmalariareport2010.pdf>.

Chapter 5

British National Formulary. 63rd edn. British Medical Association and Royal Pharmaceutical Society, 2012.

Summary of product characteristics. Depakote. eMC, 2011. <http://www.medicines.org.uk/emc/ medicine/9497/SPC/Depakote+tablets/>.

Brion, F., Nunn, A. J., and Rieutord, A. Extemporaneous preparation of oral medicines for children in European hospitals. *Acta Paediatrica* 2003; 294: 486–96.

Britten, N. Patients' ideas about medicines: A qualitative study in a general practice population. *British Journal of General Practice* 1994; 44: 465–8.

Buisson, J. Writing SOPs: Where should you start? *Pharmaceutical Journal* 2003; 271: 443–4.

Del Mar, C.B. Paul, P.G., and Hayem, M. Are antibiotics indicated as initial treatment for children with acute otitis media? A meta-analysis. *British Medical Journal* 1997; 314: 1526–9.

Department of Health. *Improving Patients' Access to Medicines: A Guide to Implementing Nurse and Pharmacist Independent Prescribing Within the NHS in England*. DoH, 2006. <http://www.dh.gov. uk/en/Publicationsandstatistics/Publications/ PublicationsPolicyAndGuidance/DH_4133743>.

Department of Health. *Optometrist Independent Prescribing*. DoH, 2008. <http://webarchive. nationalarchives.gov.uk/+/www.dh.gov.uk/en/ Healthcare/Medicinespharmacyandindustry/ Prescriptions/TheNon-MedicalPrescribingProgramme/ Optometristindependentprescribing/index.htm>.

Department of Health. *Supplementary Prescribing by Nurses, Pharmacists, Chiropodists/Podiatrists, Physiotherapists and Radiographers within the NHS in England*. DoH, 2005. <http://www.dh.gov.uk/ prod_consum_dh/groups/dh_digitalassets/@dh/@en/ documents/digitalasset/dh_4110033.pdf>.

Department of Health. Nurse and pharmacist independent prescribing changes announced. <http:// www.dh.gov.uk/health/2012/04/prescribing-change> [23 April 2012].

Donnelly, R., McNally, M., and Barry, J. Is extemporaneous dispensing really in the best interest of patients? *Pharmaceutical Journal* 2008; 280: 251–4.

General Medical Council. *Good Practice in Prescribing Medicines*. Supplementary Guidance. GMC, 2008. <http:// www.gmc-uk.org/static/documents/content/Good_ Practice_in_Prescribing_Medicines_0911.pdf>.

General Pharmaceutical Council. *Standards of Conduct, Ethics and Performance*. GPhC, 2010. <http:// www.pharmacyregulation.org/sites/default/files/ Standards%20of%20conduct,%20ethics%20and%20 performance.pdf>.

Gilmore, I. *Prescription Charges Review: Implementing Exemption From Prescription Charges for People With Long Term Conditions*. DoH, 2009. <http://www.dh.gov.uk/ prod_consum_dh/groups/dh_digitalassets/@dh/@en/@ ps/@sta/@perf/documents/digitalasset/dh_116367.pdf>.

Medicines and Healthcare products Regulatory Agency. *Medicines and Medical Devices Regulation: What You Need to Know*. MHRA, 2008. <http://www.mhra.gov.uk/

home/groups/comms-ic/documents/websiteresources/
con2031677.pdf>.

Medicines and Healthcare products Regulatory
Agency. *Medicines information: SPC and PILs. MHRA,
2012.* <http://www.mhra.gov.uk/Safetyinformation/
Medicinesinformation/SPCandPILs/index.htm>
[Accessed 17 January 2013].

Medicines and Healthcare products Regulatory Agency.
*Off-label or Unlicensed Use of Medicines: Prescribers'
Responsibilities.* MHRA, 2009. <http://www.mhra.gov.uk/
Safetyinformation/DrugSafetyUpdate/CON087990>.

National Institute for Health and Clinical Excellence.
*Medicines Adherence: Involving Patients in Decisions About
Prescribed Medicines and Supporting Adherence.* Clinical
Guideline 76. NICE, 2009. <http://www.nice.org.uk/
nicemedia/live/11766/43042/43042.pdf>.

Pharmaceutical Services Negotiating Committee. *MUR:
The Medicines Use Review and Prescription Intervention
Service.* <http://www.psnc.org.uk/pages/mur.html>
[Accessed 27 July 2012].

Pharmaceutical Services Negotiating Committee. *New
Medicine Service (NMS).* <http://www.psnc.org.uk/
pages/nms.html> [Accessed 27 July 2012].

Pharmaceutical Services Negotiating Committee. *Tips
on Standard Operating Procedures (SOPs).* PSNC, 2005.
<http://www.psnc.org.uk/publications_detail.php/85/
standard_operating_procedure_sop_top_tips>.

World Health Organization. *Adherence to Long-Term
Therapies: Evidence for Action.* WHO, 2003. <http://apps.
who.int/medicinedocs/en/d/Js4883e/>.

Chapter 6

*Designed to Care: Renewing the National Health Service in
Scotland.* Scottish Office, 1998.

Balint, M. *The Doctor, The Patient and His Illness.*
Churchill Livingstone, 1957.

Barr, H. *Interprofessional Education 1997–2000: A
Review.* Centre for the Advancement of Interprofessional
Education, 2000.

Barr, H. *Interprofessional Education: Today, Yesterday
and Tomorrow.* Learning and Teaching Support Network
for Health Sciences and Practice, 2002.

Barr, H. *Perspectives on Shared Learning.* UK Centre for
the Advancement of Interprofessional Education, 1994.

Barr, H. (Ed.) *Piloting Interprofessional Education:
Four English Case Studies.* Occasional Paper 8. Higher
Education Academy, 2007. <http://repos.hsap.kcl.ac.uk/
content/m10202/latest>.

Barr, H., Koppell, I., Reeves, S., Hammick, M., and
Freeth, D. *Effective Interprofessional Education: Argument,
Assumption and Evidence.* Blackwell, 2005.

Biley, F.C. and Smith, K.L. Following the forsaken:
A procedural description of a problem-based learning
program in a school of nursing studies. *Nursing and Health
Sciences* 1999; 1: 93–102.

Bligh, J., Lloyd-Jones, G., and Smith, G. Early effects
of a new problem-based clinically orientated curriculum
on students' perceptions of teaching. *Medical Education*
2000; 34: 487–9.

Bond, C.M. *Concordance: A Partnership in Medicine
Taking.* Pharmaceutical Press, 2004.

Borrill, C., West, M., Shapiro, D., and Rees, A. Team
working and effectiveness in the NHS. *British Journal of
Health Care Management* 2000; 6: 364–71.

Boud, D. and Feletti, G. (Eds.) *The Challenge of Problem-
Based Learning.* 2nd, revised edn. London: Kogan Page
and New York: St Martin's Press, 1997.

British Medical Association. *Interprofessional
Education: A Report by the Board of Medical Education.*
BMA, 2006.

Byrne, P. and Long, B. *Doctors Talking to Patients.* RCGP,
1976.

Carlisle, C., Cooper, H., and Watkins, C. 'Do none
of you talk to each other?' The challenges facing the
implementation of interprofessional education. *Medical
Teacher* 2004; 26: 545–52.

Centre for the Advancement of Interprofessional
Education (CAIPE). <http://www.caipe.org.uk> [Accessed
27 November 2011].

Department of Health. *Good Doctors, Safer Patients:
A Report by the Chief Medical Officer.* DoH, 2006.
<http://www.dh.gov.uk/en/Publicationsandstatistics/
Publications/PublicationsPolicyAndGuidance/
DH_4137232>.

Department of Health. *Medical Schools: Delivering
the Doctors of the Future. A report by the Chief
Medical Officer.* DoH, 2004. <http://www.dh.gov.
uk/en/Publicationsandstatistics/Publications/
PublicationsPolicyAndGuidance/DH_4075403>.

Department of Health. *Shifting the Balance of Power
Within the NHS: Securing Delivery.* DoH, 2001. <http://
www.dh.gov.uk/en/Publicationsandstatistics/
Publications/PublicationsPolicyAndGuidance/
DH_4009844>.

Department of Health. *The NHS Improvement
Plan: Putting People at the Heart of Public Services.*
The Stationery Office, 2004. <http://www.dh.gov.
uk/en/Publicationsandstatistics/Publications/
PublicationsPolicyAndGuidance/DH_4084476>.

Department of Health. *The NHS Knowledge and
Skills Framework (NHS KSF) and the Development
Review Process.* DoH, 2004. <http://www.dh.gov.
uk/en/Publicationsandstatistics/Publications/
PublicationsPolicyAndGuidance/DH_4090843>.

Department of Health. *The Regulation of the Non-
Medical Healthcare Professions: A Review by the
Department of Health.* DoH, 2006. <http://www.
dh.gov.uk/en/Publicationsandstatistics/Publications/
PublicationsPolicyAndGuidance/DH_4137239>.

Department of Health. *Working Together,
Learning Together: A Lifelong Learning Framework
for the NHS.* DoH, 2001. <http://www.dh.gov.

uk/en/Publicationsandstatistics/Publications/
PublicationsPolicyAndGuidance/DH_4009558>.

Department of Health. *Working Together: Securing a Quality Workforce for the NHS*. DoH, 1998. <http://www.dh.gov.uk/en/Publicationsandstatistics/Publications/PublicationsPolicyAndGuidance/DH_4008565>.

Diack, H.L. How to ensure shared learning becomes a reality: A report from a double agent. *Pharmaceutical Journal* 2004; 272: 702.

Diack, L. and Smith, D.F. The media and the management of a food crisis: Aberdeen's typhoid outbreak in 1964. In V. Berridge and K. Loughlin (Eds) *Medicine, the Market and the Mass Media: Producing Health in the 20th Century*. Routledge, 2004.

Diack, L., Gibson, M., Healey, T., Bond, C., and Mackenzie, H. *The Aberdeen Interprofessional Health and Social Care Initiative: Final report*. University of Aberdeen and Robert Gordon University, 2008. <http://www.ipe.org.uk>.

Freeth, D., Hammick, M., Reeves, S., Koppel, I., and Barr, H. *Effective Interprofessional Education: Development, Delivery and Evaluation*. Blackwell, 2005.

General Medical Council. *Good Medical Practice*. GMC, 2006. <http://www.gmc-uk.org/static/documents/content/GMP_0910.pdf>.

General Medical Council. *Review of Tomorrow's Doctors*. GMC, 2006.

General Medical Council. *Tomorrow's Doctors*. GMC, 1998.

General Medical Council. *Tomorrow's Doctors*. GMC, 2003.

General Pharmaceutical Council. *Future Pharmacists: Standards for the Initial Education and Training of Pharmacists*. GPhC, 2011. <http://www.pharmacyregulation.org/sites/default/files/GPhC_Future_Pharmacists.pdf>.

Glen, S. and Reeves, S. Developing interprofessional education in the pre-registration curricula: Mission impossible? *Nurse Education in Practice* 2004; 4: 45–52.

Hammick, M. Interprofessional education: Evidence from the past to guide the future. *Medical Teacher* 2000; 22: 461–7.

Horsburgh, M., Lamdin, R., and Williamson, E. Multiprofessional learning: The attitudes of medical, nursing and pharmacy students to shared learning. *Medical Education* 2001; 35: 876–83.

Kennedy, I. *Final Report: Bristol Royal Infirmary Inquiry*. HMSO, 2001. <http://webarchive.nationalarchives.gov.uk/20090811143745/http://www.bristol-inquiry.org.uk>.

Kolb, D. A. *Experiential Learning: Experiences as the Source of Learning and Development*. Prentice Hall, 1984.

Kurtz, S. M. and Silverman, J. D. The Calgary–Cambridge Referenced Observation Guides: An aid to defining the curriculum and organizing the teaching in communication training programmes. *Medical Education* 1996; 30: 83–9.

Lord Laming. *The Victoria Climbié Inquiry: Report of an Inquiry by Lord Laming*. HMSO, 2003. <http://www.

dh.gov.uk/en/Publicationsandstatistics/Publications/PublicationsPolicyAndGuidance/DH_4008654>.

NHS Employers. *Quality and outcomes framework*. <http://www.nhsemployers.org/PayAndContracts/GeneralMedicalServicesContract/QOF/Pages/QualityOutcomesFramework.aspx> [Accessed 17 January 2013].

O'Brien, S. *The Caleb Ness Inquiry: Report of an Inquiry by Susan O'Brien, QC*. Edinburgh: HMSO, 2003 <http://www.nhslothian.scot.nhs.uk/publichealth/2005/ar2003/caleb/cnr.pdf>.

Parsell, G. and Bligh, J. Interprofessional learning. *Postgraduate Medical Journal* 1998; 74: 89–95.

Parsell, G., Spalding R., and Bligh, J. Shared goals, shared learning: Evaluation of a multiprofessional course for undergraduate students. *Medical Education* 1998; 32: 304–11.

Reeves, S., Freeth, D., McCrorie, P., and Perry, D. 'It teaches you what to expect in future ...': Interprofessional learning on a training ward for medical, nursing, occupational therapy and physiotherapy students. *Medical Education* 2002; 36: 337–44.

Royal College of General Practitioners. *The Future General Practitioner*. RCGP, 1972.

Royal Pharmaceutical Society. *Promotion of Shared Learning: A Progress Report*. RPS, 1998.

Scobie, S.D., Lawson, M., Cooke, J., Cantrill, J.A., and Roberts, T.E. Multiprofessional learning between medical and pharmacy students through problem-based learning. *Pharmaceutical Journal* 1998; 261: R36.

Scottish Executive. *The Right Medicine: A Strategy for Pharmaceutical Care in Scotland*. Scottish Executive, 2002. <http://www.scotland.gov.uk/Resource/Doc/158742/0043086.pdf>.

Silverman, J.D., Kurtz, S.M., and Draper, J. *Skills for communicating with patients*. Radcliffe, 2005.

Smith, J. *The Harold Shipman Inquiry: Report of an Inquiry by Dame Janet Smith*. HMSO, 2002. <http://www.shipman-inquiry.org.uk/reports.asp>.

Stewart, D., MacLure, K., George, J., Bond, C., Diack, L., McCaig, D., and Cunningham, S. Pharmacist prescribing in primary care: The views of patients across Great Britain who had experienced the service. *International Journal of Pharmacy Practice* 2011; 19: 328–32.

Steinert, Y. *Learning Together to Teach Together: Interdisciplinary Learning and Faculty Development*. Ottawa: Health Canada, 2004.

Tate, P. *The Doctor's Communication Handbook*. 5th edn. Radcliffe, 2007.

Wanless, D. *Securing Our Future Health: Taking a Long-Term View*. The Wanless Report. HM Treasury, 2002. <http://www.hm-treasury.gov.uk/d/letter_to_chex.pdf>.

Zwarenstein, M., Reeves, S., Barr, H., Hammick, M., Koppel, I., and Atkins, J. *Interprofessional Education: Effects on Professional Practice and Health Care Outcomes*. Cochrane Library, Issue 4. John Wiley & Sons, 2003.

Chapter 7

Mental Capacity Act 2005. HMSO, 2005.

Ajzen, I. From intentions to actions: A theory of planned behavior. In J. Kuhl and J. Beckmann (Eds.) *Action-Control: From Cognition to Behavior*. Heidelberg: Springer, 1985, pp. 11–39.

Armitage, C.J., and Talibudeen, L. Test of a brief theory of planned behaviour-based intervention to change adolescent safe sex intentions. *British Journal of Psychology* 2010; 101: 155–72.

Kasl, S.V. and Cobb, S. Health behaviour, illness behaviour and sick role behaviour: ii. Sick role behaviour. *Archives of Environmental Health* 1966; 12: 531–41.

Marks, D.F., Murray, M., Evans, B., and Willig, C. *Health Psychology: Theory, Research and Practice*. Sage, 2000.

Matarazzo, J.D. Behavioural health: A 1990 challenge for the health sciences professions. In J. D. Matarazzo, N. E. Miller, S.M. Weiss, and J.A. Herd (Eds.) *Behavioural Health: A Handbook of Health Enhancement and Disease Prevention*. New York: Wiley, 1984, pp. 3–40.

Norman, P. and Brain, K. An application of an extended health belief model to the prediction of breast self-examination among women with a family history of breast cancer. *British Journal of Health Psychology* 2005; 10: 1–16.

Ogden, J., Baig, S., Earnshaw, G., Elkington, H., Henderson, E., Linsday. J., and Nandy, S. What is health? Where GPs' and patients' worlds collide. *Patient Education and Counselling* 2001; 45: 265–9.

Prochaska, J.Q. and DiClemente, C.C. Transtheoretical therapy: Toward a more integrative model of change. *Psychotherapy: Theory, Research and Practice* 1982; 20: 161–73.

Rosenstock, I.M. Why people use health services. *Millbank Memorial Fund Quarterly* 1966; 44: 94–124.

Rosenstock, I.M., Stretcher, V.J., and Becker, M.J. The health belief model and HIV risk behaviour change. In R. J. DiClemente and J.L. Peterson (Eds.) *Preventing AIDS: Theories and Methods of Behavioural Interventions*. New York: Plenum Press, 1994, pp. 5–24.

Sheikh, S. and Furman, A. A cross-cultural study of mental health beliefs and attitudes towards seeking professional help. *Social Psychiatry, Psychiatry and Epidemiology* 2000; 35: 326–34.

Wade, T.D. and Kendler, K.S. Absence of interactions between social support and stressful life events in the prediction of major depression and depressive symptomatology in women. *Psychological Medicine* 2000; 30: 965–74.

Chapter 8

British National Formulary. 63rd edn. British Medical Association and Royal Pharmaceutical Society, 2012.

Room for Review: A Guide to Medication Review: The Agenda for Patients, Practitioners and Managers. Medicines Partnership, 2002.

American College of Rheumatology. *Arthritis Impact Measurement Scales (AIMS/AIMS2)*. <http://www.rheumatology.org/practice/clinical/clinicianresearchers/outcomes-instrumentation/AIMS.asp> [Accessed 28 July 2012].

Barber, N. What constitutes good prescribing? *British Medical Journal* 1995; 310: 923–5.

Hepler, C.D. and Strand, L.M. Opportunities and responsibilities in pharmaceutical care. *American Journal of Hospital Pharmacy* 1990; 47: 533–43.

Medicines and Healthcare products Regulatory Agency. *Good pharmacovigilance practice*. <http://www.mhra.gov.uk/Howweregulate/Medicines/Inspectionandstandards/GoodPharmacovigilancePractice/Background/index.htm> [Accessed 17 January 2013].

National Institute for Health and Clinical Excellence. *Measuring effectiveness and cost effectiveness: The QALY*. <http://www.nice.org.uk/newsroom/features/measuringeffectivenessandcosteffectivenesstheqaly.jsp> [Accessed 17 January 2013].

Pharmaceutical Services Negotiating Committee. *The Medicines Use Review and Prescription Intervention Service*. <http://www.psnc.org.uk/pages/mur.html> [Accessed 17 January 2013].

Pirmohamed, M., James, S., Meakin, S., Green, C, Scott, A.K., Walley, T.J., Farrar K., Park B.K., and Breckenridge, A.M. Adverse drug reactions as cause of admission to hospital: Prospective analysis of 18 820 patients. *British Medical Journal* 2004; 329: 15–19.

Rosenberg, W. and Donald, A. Evidence based medicine: An approach to clinical problem-solving. *British Medical Journal* 1995; 310: 1122–6.

SF-36.org. A community for measuring health outcomes using SF tools. <http://www.sf-36.org> [Accessed 17 January 2013].

Index